CIRCUMCISION

CIRCUMCISION

How an Ancient Ritual
Became a Questionable Surgery—A Complete Analysis

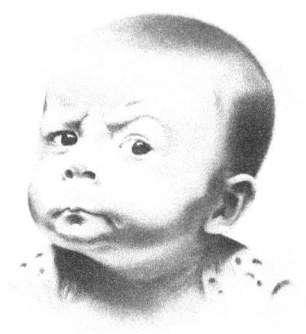

Kenneth S. Lipman, PhD

A K I V A   P R E S S

Akiva Press LLC

ISBN 979-8-9903337-0-3 (hardcover)
ISBN 979-8-9903337-2-7 (softcover)
ISBN 979-8-9903337-1-0 (ebook)
ISBN 979-8-9903337-3-4 (audiobook)

Library of Congress Control Number: 2024909162

Cover illustration by Julie Cohn
Interior illustrations by Chynna DeSimone

Contents

WHY I WROTE THIS BOOK—THIS ISN'T AS BORING AS IT SOUNDS   xi

CHAPTER ONE: CIRCUMCISION 101—THE BASICS   3

What Is The Foreskin?   3

Hygiene and Foreskin Retraction   7

Purpose of the Foreskin   7

Is the Foreskin an Organ?   8

What is Male Circumcision?   9

Prevalence of Circumcision   9

When Did Circumcision Start?   11

But Why Circumcise?   12

The Hygiene Hypothesis   13

The Sacrifice Strategy   13

The Pruning Postulate   15

Lust Buster   16

Medical Misinformation   16

Cultural Consequence   16

Summary of Circumcision Basics   16

CHAPTER TWO: RELIGIOUS CIRCUMCISION—BECAUSE HE SAID SO 18

Jewish Circumcision 18

    What Does the Torah Say about Circumcision? *19*

    Who Wrote the Torah Again? *19*

    Torah Lost and Found *22*

    Farewell to the Foreskin *29*

    The Metzitzah Miscalculation *31*

    Jewish Pushback against Metzitzah *33*

    Brit Milah—The Ceremony as It Is Performed Today *33*

    Some Jews Question the Entire Brit *36*

    Alternatives to Brit Milah *36*

    Antisemitism, Philosemitism, and Circumcision *38*

    Jewish Identity and Change *41*

    Summary of Jewish Circ *42*

Muslim Circ 43

Christian Views of Circ 45

Other Religions' Views of Circ 46

Summary of Ritual Circ 46

CHAPTER THREE: MEDICAL CIRCUMCISION, OR WHY I ATE KELLOGG'S SUGAR FROSTED FLAKES AS A CHILD 47

The History of Medical Circ 47

Medical Circ Procedure 51

Possible Benefits of Medical Circ 51

    Reduction in the Human Papillomavirus (HPV) Infection Rate *51*

    Reduction in HIV/AIDS Rate *52*

    Reduction of Sexually Transmitted Infections other than HIV *57*

    Reduction of Penile Cancer Rate *58*

    Reduction in Urinary Tract Infection Rate *59*

    Hygiene *60*

    Conformity of Appearance *60*

    Treatment of Phimosis *60*

    Treatment of Lichen Sclerosus *62*

    Mistaken Intact Attacks *62*

    Summary of Possible Benefits of Circ *63*

Harms from Circ   63

   Pain   63

   Trauma   67

   Circ Complications Overview   68

   Infections Other Than UTIs or STIs   69

   Sudden Infant Death Syndrome   70

   Bleeding   70

   Cancer   71

   Breastfeeding Disruption   71

   Lopsided Foreskin   71

   Fistulas   71

   Adhesions   72

   Corona Obliteration   72

   Necrosis   72

   Amputation   72

   Loss of Pheromones?   73

   Opioid Addiction   73

   Meatitis and Meatal Stenosis   73

   Death   74

   Curvature of the Penis   74

   Miscellaneous Possible Complications   75

   Problems Later in Life   76

Doctors' Statements   84

Medical Summary and Conclusion   85

CHAPTER FOUR: INTACT MEN AND THE WOMEN WHO LOVE THEM—FEMALE PERSPECTIVES ON MALE CIRCUMCISION   86

The Foreskin's Silken Glide   86

Friction's Flame   87

Thrust Force   87

Thrust Depth   88

Intercourse Length of Time   88

Thrust Lubrication   88

Thrust Rhythm   89

Circ and Motherhood   90

CONTENTS

CHAPTER FIVE: PENIS FACIALS ANYONE? FORESKIN FINANCES 91

Jalopies for Patients 91

Mercedes for Doctors 92

Lamborghinis for the Hospital 92

Research 93

Skin Grafts 93

Cosmetics 93

Profit from Invisible Foreskins 94

The Morality of Foreskin Sales 96

CHAPTER SIX: RIGHTS OR RITES? THE ETHICS AND LEGALITY OF CIRC 97

Circ in Court 98

Medical Associations' Views 99

CHAPTER SEVEN: THE UNKINDEST CUT—AMERICAN MEDICINE'S STUBBORN STANCE ON CIRC 102

Fear of Defying Established Guidelines 102

Clinical Detachment 104

Ignorance of Foreskin Issues 104

Change in Medicine is Difficult 105

Publication Bias 106

Fear of Being Labeled an Antisemite 106

Financial Incentives 106

Hard-to-Break Inertia 107

CHAPTER EIGHT: TOOLS OF THE TRADE—CIRC INSTRUMENTS 108

The Shield 108

The Gomco Clamp 108

The Mogen Clamp 109

The Plastibell 109

The Circular Stapler 109

PrePex 109

CONTENTS

Laser   109

Heating Cautery   110

CHAPTER NINE: CONCLUSION   112

ACKNOWLEDGMENTS   114

SELECTED BIBLIOGRAPHY OF ONLINE RESOURCES   115

ENDNOTES   117

Why I Wrote This Book

This Isn't As Boring As It Sounds

During the months my mother was pregnant with me, she faithfully drank a quart of milk daily to ensure my health. When I finally arrived, she said it was the happiest day of her life.

Yet, on my eighth day, amid a grand celebration, she allowed a mohel (Jewish circumciser) to wield a knife and sever one of my most sensitive body parts—my foreskin—without benefit of anesthesia. He then painstakingly tore off any remaining shreds with his fingernails, as is the custom.

This ceremony is called *Brit Milah* (pronounced *breet* or *bris mee-lah*)—the covenant of circumcision—and it holds profound significance in Judaism as an initiation into the community. But circumcision isn't just for Jews. Worldwide, there are three significant groups in which most of the population circumcises, listed with their estimated rates: Jews (90%), Muslims (90%), and Americans of all faiths (65%). Why Americans? We'll get to that.

It's crucial to keep in mind a distinction that comes up throughout the book: religious, or ritual, circumcision, as practiced by Jews and Muslims, is performed for religious reasons only; medical circumcision is done purely for alleged health benefits.

In the 1950s, when I was born, both doctors and mohels wrongly believed that circumcision was a painless minor surgery even though it would have been a first for medicine if a person truly didn't feel pain upon complete removal of a nerve-packed body part. Today, most circumcisions are *still* performed without effective anesthesia even when done in a hospital where it is readily available.[1]

———————

You might wonder if I'm questioning circumcision because I'm a self-hating Jew or even an antisemite. To the contrary, my lineage is woven with the threads of Jewish persecution; my parents are Holocaust survivors, my mother endured the horrors of Auschwitz. I've felt the sting of fists and the shadow of discrimination simply for being Jewish. Antisemitism isn't just an abstract concept for me; it's personal.

I attended Orthodox Jewish day schools until the age of 18 and am a steadfast Zionist. I love being Jewish. Circumcision was a cornerstone of my identity, a sacred tradition tracing back through countless generations, something I never questioned. But beginning in my thirties, I started losing sensation in my penis. This often happens to fully circumcised men, as penile areas that were never meant to be without their warm mucus sheath often become leathery over time. The process often happens so gradually that most men aren't aware of it, until perhaps they experience erectile dysfunction, which occurs at a dramatically higher rate with circumcised men. (Later on, I will go into much greater detail, and cite sources for everything I write in this brief introduction.)

I was perplexed—surely evolution, that grand sculptor, would have perfected the act of reproduction. I was compelled to unravel the mystery. Initially, I had no idea circumcision might be involved, but eventually the pieces began to fall into place. It took me many years to screw up my courage, but by 2015, I was finally able to confront the bedrock assumptions of my upbringing.

———————

A few technical notes: Generally, when I speak about circumcision, I refer to routine male circumcision, either done for religious or medical reasons and performed on a healthy penis. There are extremely rare circumstances where circumcision may be medically indicated, which I will address later, but that is not my main focus. To streamline the text and avoid repetition, I use the term "circ" to mean "routine male circumcision" and describe an uncircumcised male as "intact." Finally, female circumcision is an important topic that unfortunately falls outside the scope of this book.

Circ is the most commonly performed surgical procedure in the world,[2] and much has been written about its minutiae, such as what instruments to use, but few authors address *why* it is being done. As a United Nations report noted, "Our review of the literature [on circ] shows . . . relatively little literature on this very common surgical procedure. . . . There is a lack of a standardized operating practice for circumcision, including the management and reporting of adverse events."[3] Another study reached a similar conclusion.[4]

After analyzing books, medical journals, religious texts, videos, and my own interviews, I discovered the reason for the "relatively little literature": circ is a goalless enterprise. There's no reason to do the surgery, so it's impossible to ascertain the right technique! And there's little on "adverse events" because nobody wants to draw attention to how common they are, so they are often ignored or intentionally hidden.

In fact, not one medical organization in the world recommends circ.[5] Only the American Academy of Pediatrics (AAP) writes that "the benefits outweigh the risks," but it stops short of an official circ recommendation. Astoundingly, not one book recommends the practice either. The closest I found to an endorsement was in books penned by mohels, who were primarily focused on meticulously executing the *mitzvah* (Jewish commandment) of circ.

Few topics are as controversial as circ, which touches on sexuality, religion, money, ethnicity, and entrenched medical practice. So it's no wonder that circ is a stealth surgery that survives on inertia because most people don't want to address it. Parents who have their child circumcised in a hospital usually don't see the actual surgery, and those who attend a brit rarely directly view the procedure either. One nurse noted that young children are always treated with their parents present, often holding them, except in the case of circ.[6]

US hospitals and mohels currently don't routinely report statistics on circ, so we don't have comprehensive information on how often it's done and what the problems are. And many circumcised men are reluctant to talk about it or don't realize what they're missing since they have no point of comparison on how it feels to be intact. In general, men often have trouble talking about their vulnerabilities, especially sexual ones.[7]

Whether you're an expectant parent or a health professional, you want to make the best decision for a newborn boy. This comprehensive guide to circumcision is the only source that will cover all its aspects thoroughly, in an easily understandable way, so that you can make an informed choice.

In this book, you will learn:

- Why circumcision does not improve a baby's health
- Circumcision's significant physical and mental health risks
- Why both men and women have better sex if the man is uncircumcised
- The secret financial incentives behind the $5.7 billion circumcision industry
- Why even those who adhere to Judaism or Islam may not be required to circumcise their child

Pain alone would be reason enough to question circ, but it also can cause both immediate and lifelong problems (if you survive it—yes, it can be fatal).

I am not a medical doctor; however, an anesthesiologist, pediatrician, and urologist have checked this book for accuracy. I didn't write it to attack Jews, Muslims, doctors, or anyone else. I wrote it to thoroughly evaluate a practice that was created by some questionable judgments, made by just a small group of men, a long time ago.

CIRCUMCISION

CHAPTER ONE

Circumcision 101

The Basics

WHAT IS THE FORESKIN?

When I was growing up in Chicago, I heard that the foreskin was just "a useless flap of skin." I don't know how this pervasive idea got started, but a doctor as far away as Australia blogged that he received the same childhood message. I've read the same phrase in other places online, and it slipped into the pages of the book *Sexy Origins and Intimate Things*.[8,9] But the foreskin is not useless, not a flap, and not just skin. Calling the foreskin "skin" is as foolish as categorizing the hand as "skin" because skin envelopes it. The medical term for foreskin is prepuce, which is a better term because it transcends the skin classification, but I will use the term foreskin because I want this book to be accessible to the general reader.

The foreskin is an elegantly designed solution to a complex evolutionary dilemma. The penis must have a resilient and dry exterior to prevent unwanted adhesion to clothing and other external elements while it protrudes from the body. Yet it also must be exquisitely sensitive and moist enough to facilitate sexual pleasure within the embrace of the vagina. The solution is the insulating foreskin sheath around the penis, which is dry on the outside and lubricated on the inside so that when it unfolds upon erection, it will present a slick surface to the vagina. And voilà, here is a side view of an intact penis (Figure 1).

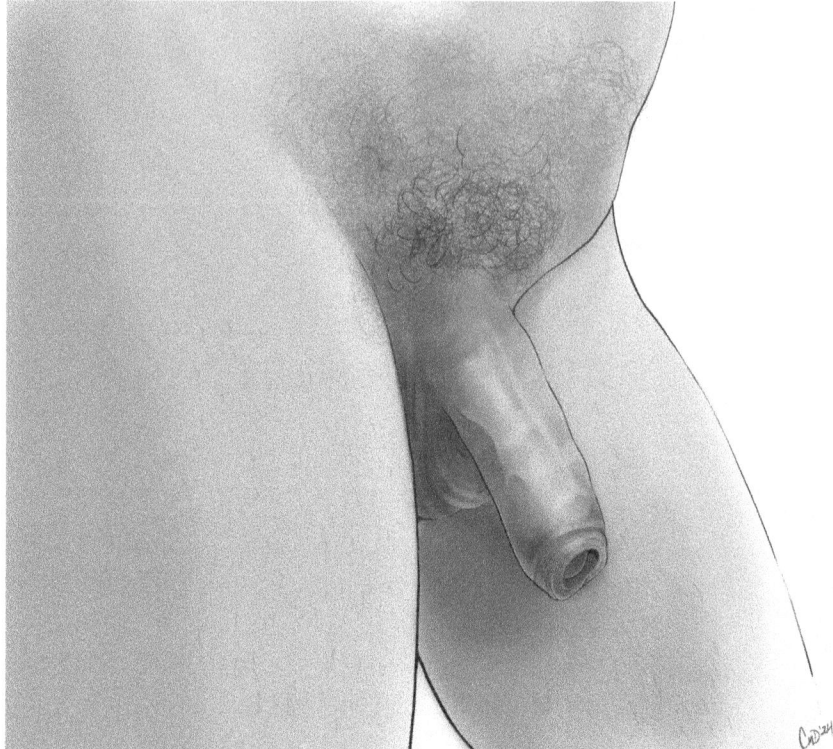

FIGURE 1. *Side view of an intact penis. Illustration by Chynna DeSimone.*

If you've never seen the whole intact apparatus, it may seem odd to you.[10]

In Figure 2, some of the important parts are labeled. Notice how the skin of the shaft and foreskin blend together at about the shaft midpoint, without an easily viewed line of demarcation. This is a significant problem in removing the foreskin that I'll discuss later. Also, note that the glans is the head of the penis. Remember that term, because it will come up a lot.

While the exterior foreskin that encases the penis is visible, you can't see the moist mucous membrane on the inside, which is lubricated by oily secretions called smegma, which keeps the glans soft. The foreskin is analogous to the eyelid, which retracts and also has a mucous membrane that keeps the eye moist.[11]

The foreskin is infused with a network of specialized nerve endings and sensory structures such as fine touch receptors (which sense pressure, touch, and

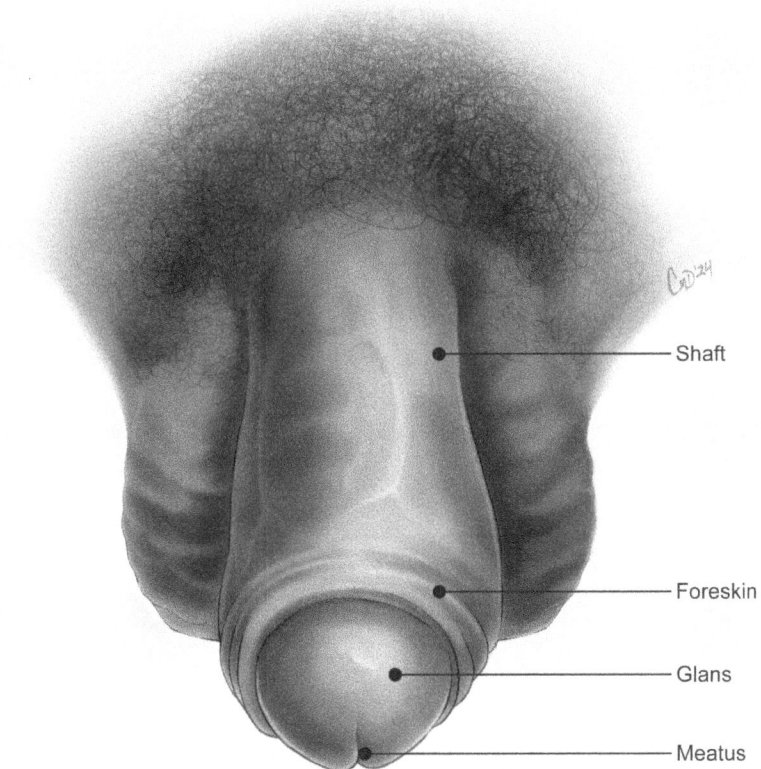

Shaft

Foreskin

Glans

Meatus

FIGURE 2. *Partially retracted foreskin of an intact man. Illustration by Chynna DeSimone.*

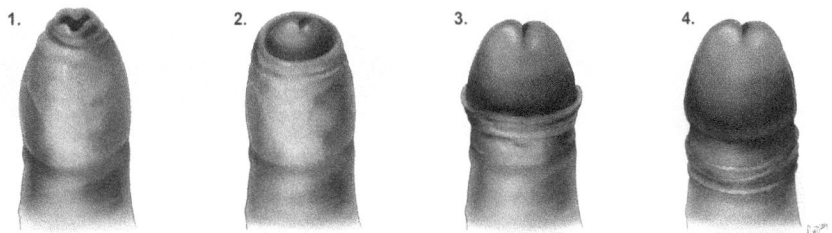

FIGURE 3. *Time series—unfurling the foreskin of an erect penis. Illustration by Chynna DeSimone.*

vibration), the most important of which are Meissner's corpuscles.[12,13] To get an idea of how these corpuscles feel, try this experiment.[14]

During erection, the foreskin turns inside out on the shaft, as depicted here in a time series (Figure 3).

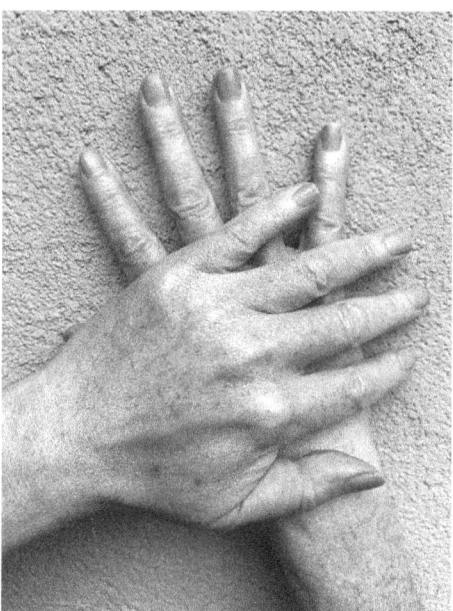

FIGURE 4. *Left hand over right hand.*

Part 1: Place your left hand over the top of your right hand, like in Figure 4.

Now run your left hand slowly over the *top* of your right hand (on a spot that doesn't have hair—that's important) and notice the sensation.

Part 2: Run your left hand slowly over your right hand's *palm*. This should feel more sensitive and enjoyable. That's because palms are suffused with Meissner's corpuscles. It is probably one reason we enjoy petting animals. Reader, would you willingly give this up? The foreskin's muscle fibers stretch during sexual intercourse, stimulating the Meissner's corpuscles.

Besides Meissner's corpuscles, the foreskin is a bundle of nerves, sweat glands, muscle, blood vessels, oil glands, and a mucous inner layer.[15] The adult foreskin is surprisingly large—if it were unfolded and laid flat, it would approximate the size of a 3-by-5-inch index card, or about 15 square inches (97 square centimeters).[16] In fact, one anticirc organization is named 15 Square.[17]

The foreskin has several erogenous zones: the frenulum, ridge mucosa, preputial orifice (where the foreskin opens), and external fold (Figure 5).

Continuous stimulation of any of these areas usually elicits orgasm and ejaculation.[18] The highest concentration of Meissner's corpuscles is where the ridged band merges with the frenulum.[19] Dr. Alfonso Cepeda-Emiliani calls this region

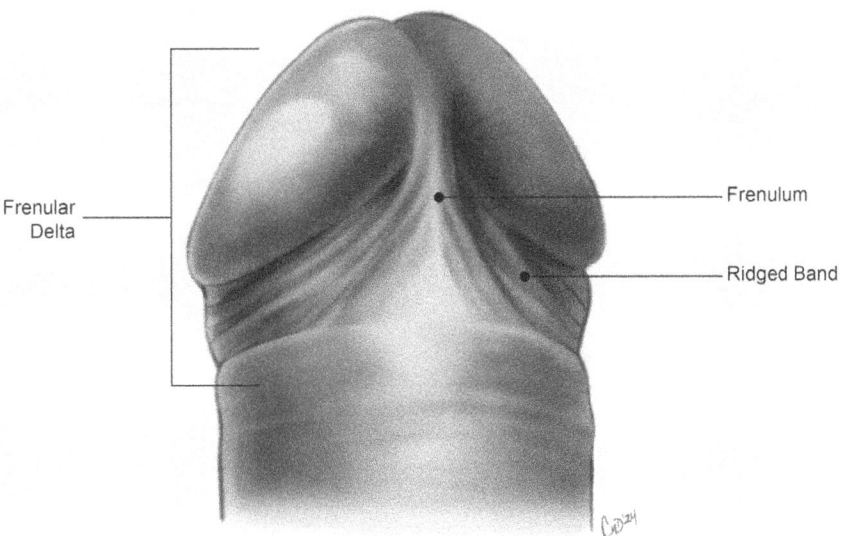

Frenular Delta

Frenulum

Ridged Band

FIGURE 5. *Frenulum and ridged band, the "frenular delta." Illustration by Chynna DeSimone.*

the frenular delta, which he says is "ground zero for sexual pleasure—the F-spot" due to the unique, dense confluence of four different nerve types.[20]

Jewish circumcision always removes the frenulum, and I grieve its loss the most. Some of the intact men I interviewed were shocked that I didn't have one and said they couldn't imagine sex without it.

Hygiene and Foreskin Retraction

At birth, the foreskin is fused to the glans, like a fingernail on a finger, blocking irritants. The glans is further protected by the regular flow of sterile urine.[21] The foreskin retracts on its own, some time before puberty. After that, cleaning it requires only running water. Regular soap should be avoided because it can irritate the foreskin. Those determined to do a more thorough cleaning can buy special gels designed for this purpose.[22]

Purpose of the Foreskin

Every male placental mammal has a foreskin;[23] in primates alone, it has existed for 65 million years.[24] Its longevity indicates that it likely has essential functions—and here is the list:[25]

Mechanical Functions

1. Protects an infant's glans from fecal matter and ammonia. In his first months, muscle fibers allow the foreskin to function as a one-way valve, preventing entry of contaminants but allowing passage of urine.
2. Shields the sensitive glans from abrasion.
3. Keeps the glans soft with smegma, an oily substance under the foreskin.[26]

Sexual Functions

1. Stokes sexual sensations during sexual intercourse when sliding up and down the shaft, by alternately covering and exposing the glans, which allows nerves time to fire and reset. After penetration, the foreskin provides a gliding action that significantly reduces friction.[27,28,29]
2. Lubricates with smegma during intercourse.[30,31]
3. Provides a vaginal seal that retains a woman's sexual fluids during intercourse.[32]
4. Contains most of a male's erotic nerve receptors.
5. Stimulates a female partner during intercourse.
6. Makes the penis look longer and thicker.

Biochemical Functions

1. Produces antibacterial and antiviral proteins such as lysozyme.[33]
2. Contains fibroblast cells that promote wound healing. (These fibroblasts are quite valuable, as we'll see in chapter 4 on foreskin finances.)
3. Contains epithelial Langerhans cells, an immune system component.[34]
4. Secretes immunoglobulins, which are antibodies against infection.[35]
5. Might emit pheromones (gases that stimulate sexual attraction).[36]

Is the Foreskin an Organ?

Intactivists are political activists who promote keeping the penis intact. They refer to the foreskin as an organ unto itself because of its special functions, vast nerve network, muscles, mucous coating, and unique ability to unfold on itself. Also, the American Academy of Pediatrics defines circumcision as the "amputation of the foreskin,"[37] which sounds like an organ elimination to me. But most doctors continue to just call it skin, not an organ, so I will defer to that majority opinion.

WHAT IS MALE CIRCUMCISION?

Male circumcision is the partial or complete removal of the foreskin.

There are different styles of circ. A "high" cut is far up the shaft, away from the glans and removing the most foreskin, whereas a "low" cut is closer to the glans. Medical circ (my abbreviation for circumcision) removes widely varying amounts of foreskin. For example, when my friend had his son circumcised in a hospital, the doctor was happy to remove any part of the foreskin that my friend wanted (which makes sense, since the procedure served no purpose).

Here are comparison illustrations of an adult circumcised penis (right) and an intact penis with foreskin completely retracted (left) (Figure 6):[38]

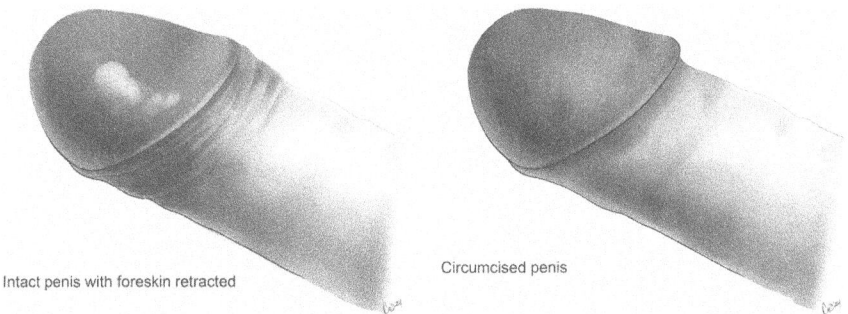

Circumcised penis

Intact penis with foreskin retracted

FIGURE 6. *Intact versus circumcised adult glans. Illustration by Chynna DeSimone.*

The intact penis has a smooth, glossy glans. The circumcised glans appears pockmarked, dried out, and weathered. It is how a man who was circumcised as an infant looks by the time he reaches his thirties.[39] Constant exposure to clothes abrades the glans, which over time fills with a hard protein called keratin, the same substance that fingernails are made of.

Ladies, which of these, if any, would you want ensconced in your vagina? More on this point later.

PREVALENCE OF CIRCUMCISION

About 39% of men worldwide are circumcised.[40] Of these, roughly two-thirds are practicing Muslims and a tiny 0.8% are Jews.[41]

Nobody records the number of Jewish or Muslim circumcisions, because they are usually private ceremonies. My best guess is that worldwide, 90% of both Jews and Muslims are circumcised.

US Circumcision Rates

The prevalence of American medical circ peaked in the 1980s at 84% and has been dropping ever since.[42] The US government hasn't calculated circ rates since 2009.

The hospital rate is estimated at 55%.[43,44,45] A 2023 map of US circ rates by state, ranging from a sky-high 91% rate in West Virginia to 10% in Nevada, is linked at the endnote.[46] However, these figures don't cover the approximate 15–20% of medical circs done at a doctor's office or those done at private religious ceremonies.

Broken down by ethnicity, here are the US rates[47]:

non-Hispanic white Americans: **91%**
non-Hispanic Black Americans: **76%**
Mexican Americans: **44%**

In 2024, I spoke with a pediatrician who practiced in California, and she said that almost all her Latino patients were intact, which contradicts the Mexican-American statistic above.

Fifteen US states saw a significant reduction in circ rates when Medicaid coverage was dropped.[48] (Medicaid is a joint federal and state program in the US that pays medical bills for people with limited finances.) All over the world, insurance coverage is one of the most significant factors in deciding whether to circumcise.

Based on these statistics, plus recent anecdotal evidence of a decline in the practice of circ, I estimate the US circ rate to be 65% in 2024.

International Circumcision Rates

Beyond American borders, circ is performed primarily in Israel; in Muslim-majority countries such as Iran, Saudi Arabia, and Somalia; within some African tribes (ranging from an 8% circ rate in Eswatini to 99.9% in Gabon);[49,50] and among some Australian and New Guinea aborigines.[51]

The prevalence of circ is under 10% in all non-Muslim Asian countries, except for South Korea, where the practice was picked up from American soldiers during the Korean War.[52] I estimate the South Korean rate at 50–60%. In the Philippines, there is a procedure called *tuli*, which involves slicing the foreskin in two, but not removing it, so it is debatable whether it should even be classified as circumcision.[53]

At the endnote is a color-coded map of each country's circ rates.[54] And the data in tabular form can be found at this endnote link.[55]

Circ Surveys

In a 2015 survey, only 31% of American doctors reported they would recommend circ when counseling parents.[56] In another 2015 US online survey, 47% of respondents said boys should be circumcised, 35% were unsure, and 17% were against.[57]

A 2021 survey for the website BabyCenter tallied responses to this question: "If you're having a boy, do you plan to have him circumcised?"[58]

Yes: **40%**　No: **54%**　Not sure yet: **5%**

Prevalence Summary

In summary, the US and South Korea are the only countries in the world with high rates of medical circ. Countries with majority Jewish or Muslim populations engage in mostly religious circ.

But how and when did circ even start?

WHEN DID CIRCUMCISION START?

Circ's origins are unknown; it likely developed independently many times. Paleolithic cave paintings have penises that are possibly missing foreskins.[59] More solid evidence of its practice is from Egyptian mummies of people who were circumcised as long as 6,000 years ago.[60] And the practice continued for centuries, because we see circ's mark on Pharaoh Amenhotep I, who reigned in the 16th century BCE.[61] (BCE is the equivalent of BC).

An Egyptian tomb's doorpost drawing from 2400 BCE (all ancient dates are approximate) depicts priests cutting two men's penises (Figure 7). The man at far left is clearly restraining the recipient, and the inscription reads: "Hold him so that he doesn't faint."[62]

One researcher, however, claims that this scenario only represents pubic hair trimming,[63] but this seems dubious.

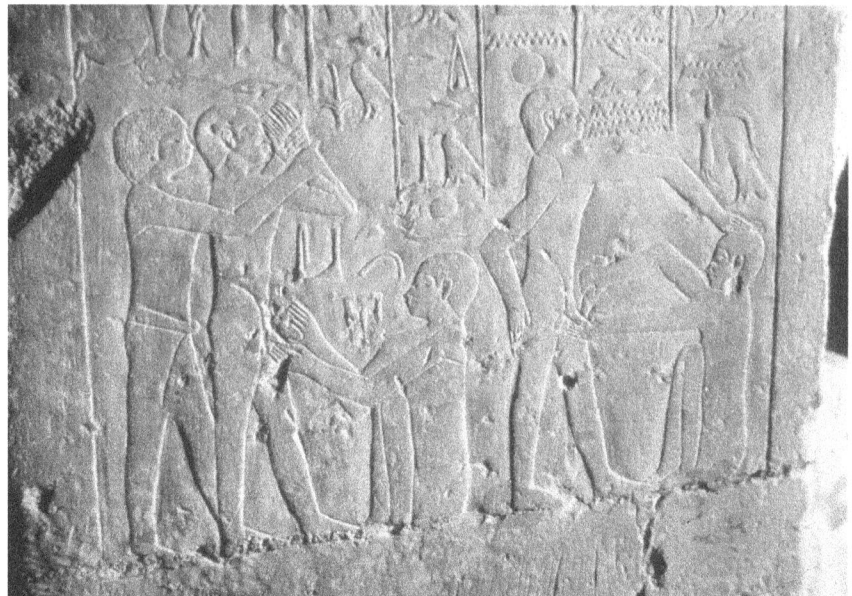

FIGURE 7. *In ancient Egypt, circumcision was depicted as a rite of passage to adulthood. This drawing of a tomb painting from Ankhmahor in Saqqara, Egypt, is the oldest known illustration of circumcision.*

The Egyptians were passionate about purity. For example, we know that Iri administered colonics as Keeper of the Pharaoh's Royal Rectum.[64] And Greek historian Herodotus observed, "Egyptians circumcise themselves, preferring to be clean rather than attractive."[65] Note how he considered the circumcised penis as uncomely. This Greek attitude would become a significant factor in the history of circ, as I'll explain later.

The Egyptian god Ra was portrayed as circumcised to signify his magnificence.[66] Throughout history, circ has been a status symbol in some circles.

We read in Jeremiah 9:24–25 (600 BCE) that various Middle Eastern tribes, such as the Edomites, Moabites, Ammonites, and, of course, Jews, also practiced circ. Perhaps these groups picked up it up from the Egyptians, or vice versa.

BUT WHY CIRCUMCISE?

Why did circ even begin? There are many theories, but the most well-known is hygiene.

The Hygiene Hypothesis

The best foreskin hygiene technique is to run warm shower water over a retracted foreskin and clean around the rim of the glans with a finger. Running water is an amenity most of us in the developed world take for granted, but in ancient times, many people didn't have it. Alternatively, they may not have known proper foreskin hygiene. Either way, not washing the area would lead to a smelly foreskin, just as not washing under your arms would create aromatic armpits. So, it may have been seen as easier simply to eliminate the foreskin.

In 1958, a Pakistani surgeon wrote, ". . . circumcision confers improved hygiene, especially to people in the lower strata of society, who water supply for bathing purposes is limited."[67]

Jewish law has always had a special focus on hygiene, prescribing handwashing before and after a meal, and washing hands and feet before entering the holy Jerusalem Temple. (Prior to 70 CE, Judaism revolved around this building. Note that CE is the equivalent of AD.) A Mishnah (the first postbiblical compilation of Jewish thought) blames one of the biblical plagues on foreskin infections.[68]

The Torah is the Jewish name for what Christians refer to as the Old Testament. (There are some textual differences, but they're not relevant to our discussion.)

Here is one Torah hygiene rule (all Torah translations in this book are mine, which I converted into modern English, skipped repetitions, and edited for readability): "One who touches a dead body shall be unclean for seven days." (Numbers 19:11)

Most farsighted was the Torah's understanding of infectivity. The Torah warns that if a man's house is contaminated with plagues, mold, and leprosy, "He shall scrape the inside of the house and place the scraped-off stuff in an unclean (off-limits) place outside the city." (Leviticus 14:45)

Philo Judaeus (20 BCE–50 CE), a Jewish philosopher, postulated a number of reasons to circumcise, and hygiene was number one: "Circumcision keeps the penis clean because no dirt can lodge under the foreskin."[69]

But there are other possible explanations for circ.

The Sacrifice Strategy

Sacrifice was important to ancient peoples. The oldest known mention is in the epic poem *Gilgamesh*, written about 4,000 years ago, which states that long life could be achieved by pleasing gods with prayer, heroism, and sacrifice.[70] The first Greek Olympics, held in 776 BCE, featured ritual sacrifices.[71] And, even in 2021, the Agnalazaha Forest residents of Madagascar would not make a conservation deal with environmentalists until they could sacrifice a cow.[72]

The Torah mentions the word "sacrifice" 234 times.[73] In particular, Jewish circ may have begun for a God who was viewed as being attached to blood as an important signifier of sacrifice.

Some examples:

- The high priest sprinkles animal blood during the Yom Kippur temple service (Leviticus 4:6).
- In the Passover story, Jews painted their doorposts with blood from a sacrificial lamb.
- Leviticus 1:5 says, "Any Israelite who wants to sacrifice shall slaughter a herd animal and fling the blood on the altar at the Tent of Meeting entrance."

As far as circ goes, it says in a midrash (a compendium of Jewish philosophy, commentary, and legends, not to be confused with the Mishnah), "Foreskin blood is sweeter to Me [God] than myrrh and frankincense."[74]

Archeologist Galit Avia Ben-Tovel believes that circ evolved in Egypt as a humane alternative to child sacrifice,[75] which was common in antiquity. Avoidance of child sacrifice is even used as an explanation for why God gave Canaan to the Jews.[76] But some Jews strayed. For example, King Hezekiah's son, Manasseh (650 BCE), "passed his son through fire." (Kings 2, 21:6)

Even today, the Ayoreo tribe of Bolivia and Paraguay buries babies alive,[77] and child sacrifice has been reported in various countries in Africa.[78]

The Divine directly demanded child sacrifice in earlier parts of the Torah, as is written,

God says, "Give me the first-born among your sons. Do the same with your cattle and flocks . . . on the eighth day you shall give it to Me." (Exodus 22:28)

"Give it to Me" is just a euphemism for murder.[79]

Also, the Torah chapter in which God commands Abraham to circumcise (in Genesis 17, which will be discussed at length later) comes shortly before

Abraham almost stabs his son Isaac as a test of his faith (Genesis 22). It seems like a strange coincidence that Abraham takes a knife to his son twice in a short period. Perhaps the two stories are actually one tale that was split over the thousands of years that it was told. Dr. David Paslin speculates that Isaac was circumcised to cure phimosis (difficulty retracting the foreskin).[80]

Circ as sacrifice was also analogized by mohel Henry Romberg, who compared circ to bringing an offering on the altar.[81] And Muslim surgeon Said Ahmed wrote that "circumcision is a sacrifice that confers profound spiritual benefits upon the parents."[82]

Similar mystical phallic associations occur today in some African locations, where every few years there is a rash of violence against sorcerers who are believed to be stealing penises. And some African tribes circumcise too.

Note that none of these sacrifices—animal sacrifice, child sacrifice, or circ—involve a personal sacrifice. This leads to what I dub the Golden Rule of Sacrifice: *Always sacrifice someone else.*

The Pruning Postulate

A Filipino doctor told me that, at age 10, he was told that he couldn't impregnate a woman unless he was circumcised. This belief may have been another ancient rationale for circ. Perhaps it seemed like the foreskin might block ejaculation, even though it retracts. Philo said it directly: Circ increases fertility, allowing "seminal fluid to proceed easily on its path."[83]

The Torah also makes an analogy between circ and fertility, "When you plant a tree, regard its fruit as foreskin. For three years it shall be uncircumcised and not eaten." (Leviticus 19:23)

And just a few verses before the circ section, God says, "I will make you exceedingly fruitful, and make you into nations, and kings will emerge from you." (Genesis 17:6)

Finally, note that God promises that Sarah will conceive in the chapter after Abraham is circumcised, which hints at a connection.

Biblical scholar Francesca Stavrakopoulou theorizes that the ancients connected circ to fertility and also to spiritual cleanliness since when a woman gives birth to a boy, she is considered spiritually unclean for seven days (Leviticus 12:2–4).[84]

But sex is about more than fertility; just ask Philo.

Lust Buster

Prolific phallic philosopher Philo wrote, "To remove lust that burdens the soul, the lawgivers ordered mutilation of the instrument which serves this."[85]

In a midrash, Rabbi Hunia says, "When a woman is intimate with an uncircumcised man, she finds it hard to tear herself away."[86] This implies that male circumcision reduces sexual pleasure for a woman too. As we shall see later, this turns out to be true.

Maimonides (1138–1204) was a prominent Jewish philosopher and medical doctor. He writes in his book *A Guide for the Perplexed*, "Circumcision counteracts excessive lust."[87]

These sentiments are repeated in modern times. Here are two quotes from Jews, in 1985:

"Foreskin represents man's worst animal-like urges and must be forcibly harnessed."—NOSSON SCHERMAN

"Impairment of sexual sensation is a special virtue of circumcision."—RABBI PAYSACH KROHN[88]

A friend commenting on my book said, "Maybe circ accounts for Jewish intellectualism and all those Nobel prizes."

Medical Misinformation

Herodotus, 400 BCE, wrote that circ prevented penile infections,[89] kicking off millennia of medical justifications for circ. Centuries later, Philo made the same claim.[90]

Cultural Consequence

The circumcised penis can be viewed as an ethnic or cultural identifier, and a measure of group solidarity. Tacitus wrote, "[Jews] circumcise to be distinguished from other people."[91]

Circ has marked Jews as different at many points in history. It consternated the ancient Greeks and was infamously used by the Nazis as a Jewish marker.

SUMMARY OF CIRCUMCISION BASICS

Circ removes foreskin areas that have important functions. There are many theories of how circ began; a combination of several of them may have contributed to the practice.

However it began, tribal leaders possibly found that the best way to promote compliance was to say that God demanded the sacrifice. This leads to the next chapter, Religious Circumcision. (If religious circumcision doesn't interest you, please skip ahead to chapter 3: Medical Circumcision.)

CHAPTER TWO

Religious Circumcision

Because He Said So

This chapter will analyze religious texts, where faith collides with foreskin. I do not intend to dismiss biblical supernatural events as "unscientific" and therefore false, for I am a spiritual person who believes that miracles are possible. I will only examine many of the text's problematic details, which seem to have become distorted over the millennia that these stories were told. Given that millions of people regard these tracts as infallible, I feel compelled to go into great detail to make my case. Let's start with Judaism.

JEWISH CIRCUMCISION

This is not the book I originally wanted to write. When I started my research, I was hoping for a title along the lines of *The Wisdom of the Torah—The Joy of Circumcision*. But alas, I have produced its antithesis. All Jews are my family, and this is dedicated to all the Jewish boys who are facing circ.

Orthodox Jews circumcise because they believe God commanded them to do so in the Torah. It is a core belief of Orthodox Judaism, that God dictated the first five Torah books to Moses at Mount Sinai (1312 BCE), and every word has been faithfully transmitted since that time with no changes.[92]

What Does the Torah Say about Circumcision?

Let's examine the text of Genesis, chapter 17, (2000 BCE). This is the only section of the Torah that commands Jews to circumcise.

17:1—Yahweh said to Abram, "I am Almighty God."

17:5—"Your name is no longer Abram, but rather Abraham, for you will father a multitude of nations." (One explanation for this is that the "h" is added as one letter of Yahweh, to symbolize Abraham's divine connection.)

17:7—"I will establish between you and your descendants an everlasting covenant."

17:8—"I will give them the entire land of Canaan as a permanent possession, and I will be to them as Elohim." (Notice that God's name has gone from Yahweh to Elohim.)

17:10–12—"At eight days old, every male among you, including your slaves, shall circumcise the flesh of his foreskin, as a symbol of our covenant."

17:14—"A male who does not circumcise shall be excommunicated."

17:15—And Elohim said to Abraham, "Do not call your wife Sarai, for Sarah is her name." (Sarah gets an "h" added as well.)

———————

This description of the circ covenant seems clear "cut," but it isn't. To begin with, notice that in verse 5, God changes Abram's name. The natural follow-up would be to change Sarai's name, but that doesn't happen until verse 15. Also, the initial verse calls God "Yahweh," but then verse 8 and onward calls him "Elohim." Yahweh was an early Hebrew name for God, and Elohim was an appellation that appeared much later in history. So it seems that a later author inserted the circ verses between the two "renaming" verses (5 and 15), and then rewrote the Sarah verse at the end, changing the name of the Divine from Yahweh to Elohim.

To understand how all this came about, we must step beyond the realm of Orthodox Judaism and consider the perspectives of biblical scholars.

Who Wrote the Torah Again?

Why would one question that Moses wrote the Torah? Because it's filled with contradictions. Richard Elliot Friedman, in his remarkable book *Who Wrote the*

Bible?, points out many biblical events that occur out of order in time and place, for example Moses going to the Tabernacle before it was even built.[93]

There is a sea of duplicated narratives within the Torah. Some examples:

- The Garden of Eden story
- Abraham's claim that his wife is his sister
- Moses getting water from a rock
- The death of King Saul
- Most importantly for our purposes, multiple versions of God's covenant with Abraham

The versions all have different details. For example, the laws in Deuteronomy conflict with the laws before it, with different lists of unkosher animals.[94]

There are even three versions of the Ten Commandments: Exodus 20:2–17, Deuteronomy 5:6–21, and Leviticus 19 (where they are embedded in a much larger list of laws).

Some biblical plots are repeated with changing casts. For example, there are suspiciously similar stories of Egyptian palace intrigue interwoven with cases of mistaken identity in three different periods: Abraham (2000 BCE),[95] Joseph (Abraham's great-grandson, 1900 BCE),[96] and Moses (1300 BCE).[97] (Further explanations are at the last three endnotes). And some of the plagues visited upon the pharaoh preceding the Jewish exodus from Egypt, are also thrown into the saga of Abraham's visit to Egypt some 600 years earlier (Genesis 12:17), further indicating that this is one story that evolved into three over time.

Then there are problematic passages like Deuteronomy 34:10: "And there was never another prophet like Moses again." This obviously was not written by Moses, as Orthodox tradition has it.

Let me introduce Rashi, considered by Orthodox Jews to be the most authoritative biblical commentator. As a child, my first inkling that something was amiss was a statement by Rashi that there is no chronological order in the Torah.[98]

There are also external incongruities to the text. For example, here's Genesis 24:11—"And Abraham's servant made the camels kneel beside the well at the time the maidens draw water." The problem with this? Abraham lived around 2000 BCE,[99] when beasts of burden were usually donkeys and never camels. For example, in the biblical story of Joseph (1500 BCE) they used donkeys. Camels weren't domesticated until about 750 years after Abraham, around 1200 BCE.[100]

Another out-of-time passage mentions forging iron (Genesis 4:22), which wasn't invented until hundreds of years later.[101]

Of course, there is archeology that is consistent with the Torah too. For example, from the period shortly after the exodus from Egypt, we have carved writings, which mention Israel and several of its still extant cities, such as Jerusalem and Ashkelon.[102] However, the question is whether we can trust any one passage, such as the one where circ is commanded.

Finally, the Hebrew used in various Torah chapters comes from different eras. Hebrew changed over time, just as any language does. Consider, for example, how much English has changed in the approximately 400 years since Shakespeare.

What can we conclude from these problems? Different versions of stories, written in varying forms of Hebrew, with changing names for God, are strong indications of more than one author. This is called the "documentary hypothesis," which holds that the Torah is a mosaic of different texts that were compiled over a span of 600 years, beginning around the 10th century BCE. Scholars use the letters J, E, D, and P to represent four hypothesized primary authors.[103]

For our purposes, we will focus on only two authors: J, the first author, and P, the last.

J got his call letter because of the name he gave God: Jehovah (the German version of Yahweh, or יהוה in Hebrew). Bloom and Rosenberg believe that J wrote the earliest version of the Torah in about 922 BCE and was part of the court of King Rehoboam of Judah (son of King Solomon).[104]

P stands for the Jewish Priestly source, and he refers to God as El or Elohim. You're probably not used to hearing the words "Jew" and "priest" in the same sentence, but the rabbinical system that Jews use today only began after the destruction of their Second Temple in 70 CE. Before that, Jewish religious leaders consisted of two types of priests: Cohens who descended from Aaron, and Levites, from the tribe of Levy. Their primary duties were performing rituals in the Holy Temple. P was a Cohen or Levy.

Most scholars believe P wrote his version in exile in Babylonia (which encompassed parts of present-day Iraq, Iran, and Syria), between 550 and 500 BCE, although some place him as early as the eighth century BCE.[105]

We can see the different ways the authors wrote, in the two versions of the Garden of Eden story that appear at the Torah's beginning. The creation of woman is an example:

Genesis 2:22–23 is written by J (I'm going to give the traditional translation first):

> **2:21**—Yahweh caused a deep sleep to fall upon the man, and took one of his ribs,
>
> **2:22**—and built the rib into a woman.

We know this is J because of the Yahweh reference. And here is P's version in Genesis 1:27, which appears in the chapter before J's rendition, "So Elohim created man in his own image; male and female he created them."

The two stories clearly differ: in J's version, woman is created from man's rib, whereas in P's version, no rib is mentioned. Even as a child, I wondered what had happened to the rib. This is my take on these verses: there is no literal reference to a "rib." The Hebrew word in the text is צלע (side). So, here is the literal translation (Genesis 2:21–22):

> **2:21**—God caused a deep sleep to fall upon the man, and took one of his sides,
>
> **2:22**—and built the side into a woman.

The Torah often speaks in euphemisms, so I speculate that "side" here refers to the penis bone (whose medical name is baculum). People of that time believed that all natural phenomena came from some divine plan. All male placental mammals, other than humans, have a penis bone. I believe J was trying to solve two biological mysteries with one divine explanation: How was woman created, and why is man missing a penis bone? J's intent was to say that Yahweh created woman from Adam's penis bone, and that is why human males don't have one. For the science on penis bones, see the endnote.[106]

Torah Lost and Found

As mentioned, Orthodox Judaism maintains that Moses wrote the original Torah, which is the same as the version that we have today. That implies that the Israelites schlepped a master copy through all their travels. This may not seem unusual to modern ears, because the Torah book we use today is the same everywhere—but that is because of the printing press. (We still have Torah scrolls today too, for liturgical use in the synagogue.) Originally, the Torah was written on five separate scrolls crafted from reed-based papyrus; later versions used animal skins. All these fragile organic materials have a limited life span. Only in the third century CE did a single giant scroll of the first five books become prevalent. There is never a mention in the Torah or anywhere else that there was a definitive set of scrolls. As Harvard Professor David Stern bluntly puts it, "There is almost no evidence for the existence of single scrolls containing the entire Pentateuch [first five Torah books]."[107]

Rabbi Aryeh Wolbe has postulated a "chain of unbroken Torah transmission" from Moses to the present day, where he lists out every single person who has held the "master copy."[108] However, I can find no evidence to support what he says. The Mishnah only gives this vague statement, "Moses received Torah from Sinai and gave it to Joshua, who gave it to the Elders, the Elders to the Prophets, and the Prophets gave it over to the Men of the Great Assembly."[109]

When the First Temple was established, in 832 BCE, some scrolls were kept there; however, it was destroyed in 586 BCE.

And according to the Torah itself, some scrolls may have been occasionally lost. For example, Kings 2 22:8 (620 BCE) says:

Hilkiah the high priest said to Shaphan the scribe, "I have found the Scroll of the Law [Torah scroll] in the house of the Lord," and Hilkiah gave the scroll to Shaphan, and he read it.

Rashi comments that the scrolls had been "hidden under a layer of stones." Things hadn't improved much some 170 years later. Here is the biblical Book of Nehemiah, chapter 8 (450 BCE):

8:1—Everyone gathered in the square and told Ezra to bring the scroll of the Law of Moses.

8:2—Ezra the priest brought the Law and

8:3—read from first light until midday, and the people were attentive.

8:9—Then Nehemiah and Ezra and the Levites said, "This day is holy to God; neither mourn nor weep," for the people were weeping when they heard the words of the Law.

Rashi explains the weeping was "because they didn't uphold the Torah properly." This implies that Ezra's readings were new information to the people, which is understandable, since many Jews had been exiled in 586 BCE and may not have had access to the scrolls. Another possibility is that Ezra rewrote the scrolls to his liking, an argument made in *Who Wrote the Bible?* Many scholars agree with this and consider Ezra the major redactor (editor) who combined all the various texts together to become the Torah. Whoever it was, it is an open question as to why he included so many repetitious or conflicting narratives. A modern editor would probably have chosen the most likely version and discarded the rest. Perhaps he thought at least one version was the true word of God, and since he didn't know which one it was, he included everything he had.

About 125 years after Ezra, a landmark version of the Torah was written. The Greek king Ptolemy II Philadelphus (309–246 BCE) was an enlightened ruler who wanted to read the Torah. He was a stickler for accuracy and had 70 scribes each independently translate the Torah into Greek. Then the versions were compared, and one final manuscript was created, which became known as the Septuagint (from the Latin *septuaginta*, literally "seventy"). It was famous in that era and the story was recounted by both the historian Josephus and the Talmud (the second major book of Jewish thought, which expands on the Mishnah). However, historian Harry Freedman convincingly argues that the account of its construction is "nothing more than a fable," and instead, a Greek-speaking non-Jewish Egyptian likely wrote it.[110] No matter how it was written, it remains an important source of knowledge about the original Torah. Judaism, however, rejects it because of some textual differences, but Christians preserve it.

The Septuagint also contains the first two Books of Maccabees, and the book of Jubilees (150 BCE), which were rejected from the Jewish biblical canon, but were accepted by some Christian denominations. These books are pertinent to our story, as I will explain later.

Next in the Torah's historical timeline are the Dead Sea Scrolls, discovered in Israeli caves and dated variously from 408 BCE to 318 CE.[111] The earliest of these scrolls overlap with the Septuagint. The scrolls are full of erasures and cross-outs, and says Stern, " . . . show that as late as the first century CE, the biblical text remained in flux."[112] The scrolls contradict one another[113] and our present day Torah too.[114]

Why don't the different versions match?

For one, intentional changes to the Torah happened throughout history. For example, the current Torah says that Goliath (the giant that David slew with a slingshot) was "6 cubits and a span." (Samuel 1, 17:4) That is 9 feet, 10 inches (about 3 meters)! But the historian Josephus and two earlier Torah versions (the Septuagint and the Dead Sea Scrolls) all have Goliath's height as "4 cubits and a span,"[115] which is a much more believable 6 feet 9 inches (about 2.1 meters). Possibly some scribe wanted to enhance David's legend by increasing the giant's height.

Another issue is accidental scribal error. It is inconceivable that a manuscript being copied and recopied over many centuries would be free of mistakes.

For example, in Isaiah 34:11, Isaiah predicts the devastation of the land of Edom: "Pelican and owl shall inherit it." The biblical Hebrew word for owl is קפוד (pronounced *kee-pode*), and even if you can't read Hebrew (which is written right to left), you can see that it is four letters. Rashi, who lived in France, confirms that "keepode" means owl and even gives the 11th century French word for it—*chouette* (which is the current French word too. In modern Hebrew, however, "keepode" means hedgehog.) Four verses later, in verse 15, we have a reference to an animal קפוז (pronounced *kee-poze*). What is "keepoze?" Bible buffs are baffled, as there are no references to it anywhere else.[116] But Rashi simply explains that "keepoze" is קפוד (keepode), the aforementioned owl. Possibly because the last letters of the two words look very similar (ד vs. ז), the scribe goofed and wrote "keepoze," instead of "keepode." Or maybe he correctly wrote a ד, but the ink faded or smeared, and later scribes interpreted it as ז.

Boredom is another unrecognized scribal problem, which inevitably introduced mistakes. Medieval scribes would frequently scribble complaints in the margins of books as they tediously copied them. For example, "As the harbor is welcome to the sailor, so the last line is to the scribe."[117]

Over the centuries many obvious errors were introduced to the Torah. However, in Talmudic times (500 CE) rabbinical authorities decided to keep the text as is.[118] Similar mistakes accrued in the Septuagint.[119]

Another confounding factor is that rabbinic law dictates that a Torah scroll cannot contain vowels or punctuation (but they are allowed today in Torah books). (Modern Hebrew usually doesn't use vowels either.) This can be confusing because the same set of consonants can mean different things depending on assumptions about what the vowels are. Early scrolls were even more difficult to decipher because they didn't even contain spaces between words; that was a later invention.[120]

So, who wrote the definitive Torah in use today? Jacob ben Chaim, in 1524, in Venice, Italy. Daniel Bomberg hired him to create a book (instead of a scroll) of the Torah. Ben Chaim wrote, "I polished the texts unto silver and gold."[121] Then they were processed by a brand new technology: the printing press.

Before this edition, there were hundreds of medieval Torah manuscripts, dating back to 800 CE, and no two agreed on every detail, something that Maimonides noted in the 12th century.[122] But once everyone in the world had the same printed book in hand, it became the standard.

Now that we understand the Torah's variants, let's look at the two primary sections regarding God's initial covenant with the Jewish people. The first is the earliest version. It's in Genesis 15, calls God Yahweh, and is therefore written by J:

15:7—"I am Yahweh, Who brought you from Ur of the Chaldees, to give you this land to inherit."

15:8—Abram said, "How will I know I inherit it?"

15:9—He replied, "Take [sacrifice] for me three heifers, three goats, three rams, a turtle dove, and a young bird."

15:10—On that day, Yahweh formed a covenant with Abram, saying, "I give this land to your descendants, from the river of Egypt until the Euphrates River."

In J's version of events, God makes a covenant with the Jewish people, and circ is never mentioned. God requires only animal sacrifice. Contrast this with Genesis 17, which we have already seen. It appears just two chapters later, and again speaks of the covenant with Abra(ha)m, but this time adds in circ. J wrote the first verse, which mentions the covenant, but P wrote the circ verses, leaving his telltale reference to God as Elohim.[123,124]

I'll cite just an abbreviated version of the key verses:

17:9-10—Elohim said to Abraham, "You and your descendants shall keep my covenant that all males shall be circumcised."

17:11—"Circumcision is a sign of the covenant between us."

In P's version, circ is an integral part of God's covenant with the Jews.

Now Jews take their contracts seriously, even if they're with supernatural beings. For example, some important concepts in common Western tort laws were first developed in the Talmud. Perhaps that is why there are so many Torah mentions of the covenant—likely written by other authors. But none of them mention circ. Here are three examples:

- **Exodus 6:4**—I established My covenant with them to give them the land of Canaan.
- **Leviticus 26:9**—I will make you fruitful and increase you, and I will set up My covenant with you.
- The entire **Deuteronomy chapter 28** describes all the details of the bargain between God and his people, and concludes, "These are the words of the covenant."

In a later era than the Five Books of Moses, the book of Joshua mentions circ, which I will discuss later. But the word covenant isn't used there either.

So it seems likely that circ's connection to the covenant was solely P's idea, as no other author cites it. As mentioned, he lived in exile in Babylonia (where the famous psalm *By the Rivers of Babylon* was written). What motivated him to put quill to parchment and insert the circ commandment?

Picture poor priest P. He lost his job, his Temple, his land, his home, and undoubtedly many friends and family when Babylon invaded. The Temple had been a pilgrimage center where thousands of Jews would gather for the major festivals, and it might have seemed impossible to practice Judaism without it[125] since rituals are vital for group bonding.[126] P might have also been frightened by the Babylonians, who didn't practice circ, and who "seize infants to dash against the rocks," as it says in the psalm. A new portable ceremony was needed, ASAP.

Maybe P believed circ would do the trick, so he penned in a divine legend—it was common in earlier times for people to write their own version of biblical events; for example, we find many of these in the Dead Sea Scrolls. Or perhaps he created Elohim's commandment as an explanation for the circ folk custom, just as J may have done with the penis bone myth. We'll never know which explanation is correct, but the result of P's actions possibly led to the world's longest-running unnecessary surgery.

P was a man of few words and leaves us no instruction as to how much foreskin to remove. Note that the biblical commandment is only to circumcise the "flesh" of the foreskin, which implies that the complete foreskin was not involved.

There is also evidence in the Book of Joshua that it was only a small amount of foreskin that was nicked ceremonially, primarily for use as a cultural marker and status symbol. Consider these verses from chapter 5:

5:2—Yahweh said to Joshua, "Make sharp knives, and circumcise again the children of Israel a second time."

5:3-4—Joshua did so, because all the men who escaped Egypt had died in the desert afterwards.

5:5—Those men were circumcised, but the men born in the wilderness were not.

5:7—So Joshua circumcised their children.

5:9—Yahweh said, "Today I removed the reproach of Egypt from you."

Although the reference to Yahweh indicates that J wrote the original text, we can see evidence that other authors amended it, since the final narrative doesn't even make sense. First God commands the Jews to circumcise a second time in verse 2, and then he explains they weren't even circumcised the first time after wandering in the desert. What is going on here?

In an incisive analysis, Rabbi David Frankel has offered the most likely explanation: In the original text, written by J, it was Joshua, not God, who encouraged the Israelites to circumcise. Later emendations by P, and possibly others, awkwardly tried to explain why the Israelites hadn't been circumcised in the first place.[127]

Also, verse 9, which says, "I removed the reproach of Egypt," lends credence to the theory that circ was a status symbol and not part of a covenant.

Finally, let's look at what Rashi says about verse 2 when it says to circumcise a second time. "'The second time' refers to the uncovering of the corona (the rim at the base of the glans) at circumcision, in other words splitting the membrane (which is part of the inner foreskin) and pulling it back, which Abraham was not commanded to do." (Later, we'll see why Rashi says this.)

In the beginning, circ may have just been a small symbolic slice, but eventually the infant's entire acroposthion, or overhang of the foreskin beyond the glans, was removed.

The acroposthion contains the smooth muscle tissue that pushes the foreskin forward and keeps it contoured to the glans. Without the acroposthion, as the circumcised boy matures, the remaining foreskin detaches from the glans and often rests behind it. The result is that after puberty the penis takes on a loosely cut appearance, and the glans is permanently exposed.[128] This display custom led to a disastrous chain of events.

Farewell to the Foreskin

In 338 BCE, Alexander the Great swept through the area that encompasses modern-day Israel. As conquerors go, Alex and his first few successors behaved decently toward the Jews. His modus operandi everywhere was to honor local practices (albeit with the unfortunate odd massacre here and there) while slowly seducing the populace with the glories of Hellenism (Greek culture). He even had a cordial meeting with the Jewish high priest in the Second Temple in Jerusalem.[129,130]

Greece was the superpower of its day, possessing renowned intellectual traditions plus a 3000-mile-long empire. Thus, Hellenism was attractive to some of my tribe.

The Greeks famously built gymnasiums where they exercised nude. In fact, the word "gymnasium" comes from *gymnos*, meaning "naked." Gymnasiums were like our cafés, where men socialized and did business.[131] So it was important for Jews who sought entrée into Greek society to pop into the gymnasium. That is where a significant cultural collision occurred.

Until then, Jews saw circ, which was practiced by many Middle Eastern groups, as normal. However, in Greek culture, circ was unknown, and in the gymnasium, displaying the glans was taboo, because it indicated sexual arousal. Thus a naked circumcised Jew was a walking defiance of Greek norms.[132] Philo observed both Greeks and Romans laughing scornfully at circumcised men.[133]

Some Jews created a way to become socially acceptable: stretch the foreskin that's left so that it covers the whole penis, which then looks uncircumcised. Many used a *Pondus Judeaus* (Jewish weight) tied to the foreskin, which over time stretched it enough to cover the entire glans. Another method, called epispasm, consisted of pulling the foreskin forward and then chemically burning it so that the scar tissue fused it to the glans.[134]

These solutions, called foreskin restoration, were largely cosmetically successful. With their reconstructed manhood, Jews even performed in the Olympics, which was a nude event.[135]

This new practice enraged the Jewish Hasmonean family, called Maccabees (hammerers) because of their fierce activism. As reported in the Book of Maccabees 1, chapter 1, written by an anonymous Jewish author in the Maccabees' voice:

1:14—Jews built a Jerusalem gymnasium in the heathen custom [meaning nudity].

1:15—And made themselves uncircumcised, abandoning the holy covenant.

The Book of Jubilees, chapter 15, reports the Maccabees' reaction:

1:33—The children of Israel don't circumcise according to the law.

1:34—There will be great wrath against them, and no forgiveness for this eternal error.

The Maccabees brought the hammer down: they forcibly circumcised every Jewish boy they found with a foreskin and recircumcised everyone who had tried to reverse their circ.[136]

Soon after, benevolent Greek rule ended. In 167 BCE, the Greek ruler Antiochus desecrated the Temple in Jerusalem, installing an image of Zeus and sacrificing pigs on the altar, and he prohibited circ.[137] Two women who had circumcised their sons had their infants bound to them and were thrown off the top of a wall.[138] Eventually, the Maccabees overthrew Antiochus (the Hanukkah story).

For some years there was peace, until Roman General Pompey conquered Jerusalem in 63 BCE, bringing new oppressors. Various revolts occurred through 132 CE. Finally, Roman Emperor Hadrian embarked on genocide, killing 580,000 Jews. Many more died of disease and starvation. Percentagewise, he killed more Jews than the Nazis. Most survivors were enslaved, but some remained in Israel, while others were once again exiled to Babylonia, just as in 587 BCE. There they created the massive 66-volume Babylonian Talmud, which became a critical source for *halacha* (Jewish law, both religious and civil).

Once again, with the loss of their land, their culture, and their (Second) Temple, the Jews were bereft. One additional pressure was early Christians' rejection of circ (more on this later).[139]

Jewish authorities particularly wanted to stop foreskin restoration. An unknown person came up with an extreme solution: a circ procedure called *periah*,[140] or "the uncovering,"[141] which involves stripping off 100% of the foreskin and its inner mucosal lining by using a sharp instrument, and/or even fingernails.

After periah, it would be exceedingly difficult to make the penis look uncircumcised (though some persistent men have had small benefits from trying to stretch shaft skin, but it takes years of effort). This is what Rashi meant when he interpreted the second circumcision in Joshua as "uncovering the corona and splitting the membrane and pulling it back." That is, they did periah. I believe that Rashi was trying to justify periah by claiming it was part of the Joshua story, even though it was centuries before periah was invented.

The tragic dialectic that has played out over the ages is that attacks on circ often only induced Jews to double down on the practice. So, in 140 CE, Jewish religious arbiters mandated periah as essential. From then on, Brit Milah meant periah.

Here are some comments of Jewish sages of that time, revealing their fixation on periah and circ as the ultimate practice:

- "He who restores his foreskin must be recircumcised, even four or five times if necessary."[142]
- "If one does not fully expose the corona [the ridge of the glans] by splitting the foreskin's membrane [periah], it is as though he has not circumcised."[143]
- "Foreskin is more unclean than all unclean things . . . a blemish above all blemishes."[144]
- One of the foremost postbiblical Jews, Rabbi Yehuda HaNasi (the chief editor of the Mishnah) upped the divine ante even more, "If not for circumcision, God would not have created the world."[145]

Thus, Jews became the first, and still only, culture that mandates radical periah, eliminating the entire sheath that preserves the penis and promotes sexual pleasure. In chapter 3, I will delineate the significant lifelong problems that this can create.

A Jewish physician I spoke with referred to periah as "horrible." Yes it is. But the story just gets worse.

The Metzitzah Miscalculation

Periah was effective at preventing attempts to reverse circ, but inadvertently created another problem.

Compare these two illustrations. The top one is of an intact penis (with the foreskin slightly retracted), and the bottom one is of a circumcised penis via periah.[146]

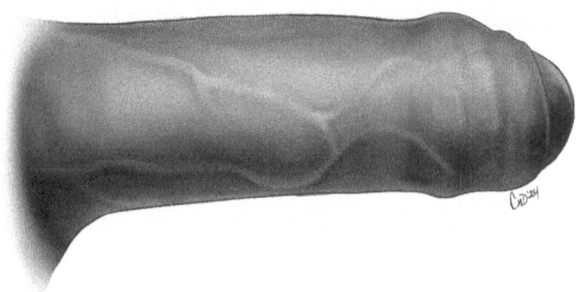

FIGURE 8. *Intact erect penis with prominent veins. Illustration by Chynna DeSimone.*

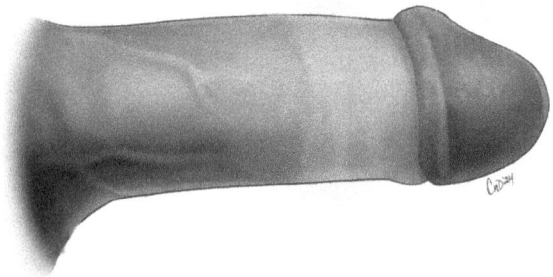

FIGURE 9. *Circumcised erect penis via periah, with a lot of missing veins. Illustration by Chynna DeSimone.*

In Figure 8, note the prominent veins of the intact penis. In Figure 9, the circumcised penis has a discolored area where the foreskin and its vein network used to be.

So, when a mohel removes the dreaded foreskin, blood drips out of the shorn shaft. What to do? Someone hit upon a solution. Are you sitting down? The mohel would suck all the blood into his mouth.

The procedure is called *metzitzah*, Hebrew for sucking, or *metzitzah b'peh* (sucking with the mouth). Metzitzah is likely based on a Hellenistic view of medicine, whereby saliva was (erroneously) seen as sterile—it would be many centuries before the discovery of the germ theory of disease.[147]

Jewish authorities embraced this technique and soon made it just as mandatory as periah, as stated in authoritative Jewish law books such as the Mishnah[148] and Talmud.[149] One prominent Talmudic sage proclaimed, "A surgeon who does not perform metzitzah is dangerous and should be removed from his post."[150] Centuries later, Maimonides echoed this.[151]

Of course, today we know that infectious diseases can be transmitted by metzitzah, most commonly, herpes simplex, but even HIV (human immunodeficiency virus, the cause of AIDS) is a risk.[152]

By the Middle Ages, the bloody circ ceremony caused some Christians to associate circ with violence, fomenting mistrust towards Jews. They reasoned: *If they're willing to do this to their own children, what would they do to ours?*[153] But as some Christians recoiled from circ, Jews latched on to it as a holy identifier.[154]

Jewish Pushback against Metzitzah

In 1831, Philipp Wolfer, a German-Jewish doctor, condemned metzitzah. In 1873, there was a documented case of sickness due to metzitzah.[155] With the health risks now more evident, in 1888, Rabbi Samson Raphael Hirsch, an important innovator who argued for more liberal practice within Jewish Orthodoxy, proposed a safer approach. He issued a halachic ruling that metzitzah could be performed using a glass tube, which is placed over the circ site. The mohel suctions the blood through the glass tube with no direct physical contact with the penis, thus eliminating the chance of infection.[156] More than 99% of all mohels today use this method, and the influential Rabbinical Council of America endorses it.[157]

However, certain fringe sects of Hasidic Jews, which constitute less than 1% of world Jewry, continue metzitzah by direct mouth-to-penis contact.[158] As I write this, a headline just appeared in *The Jewish World*: "Four New York City infants have contracted herpes from . . . metzitzah."[159] Similar articles over the years are linked in the endnotes.[160,161,162,163] The New York City Board of Health passed a law in 2012 requiring parents to sign a consent form before having their child undergo metzitzah b'peh. But, in 2015, the mayor of New York, Bill de Blasio, ended this requirement after Hasidic leaders agreed to help identify and isolate any mohels found responsible for an infection.[164] However, accountability is difficult. For example, here's a 2017 headline from the Jewish Telegraphic Agency: "Orthodox families won't identify circumcisers who gave babies herpes, NYC health spokesman says."[165]

Brit Milah—The Ceremony as It Is Performed Today

Brit Milah, or simply brit (also spelled bris), is the Jewish circ ceremony, performed on a boy's eighth day.

For those who are interested in the details, the book *Bris Milah*, by Orthodox Rabbi Henry Romberg, describes its intricacies. As is common with Orthodox Judaism, the book delineates mitzvah minutiae. For example, he discusses pinning down the exact moment of birth to guarantee that the brit will occur precisely on the eighth day, as the Torah commands.[166]

The brit is a festive event, often held at a synagogue hall or a private home. First, prayers are recited. In the Orthodox ceremony, *kvatters*, usually a married couple, take the infant from the mother and place him on a designated chair, called the Chair of Elijah. Someone lifts the baby from the chair and hands him to the father. The father then places him on the lap of someone who is designated as the *sandek*, a position of honor. Some Conservative and Reform mohels use a circumstraint, a form-fitted basket that restrains the boy from moving.[167]

There are three major parts to the Orthodox brit ceremony:

1. Chituch—Cutting the Foreskin

Some mohels then cut a dorsal slit in the foreskin with a scalpel (knife). However, this method risks harming the glans. Thus, an unknown inventor created a penile shield for Jewish circ, the first known mention of which was in 1580.[168] The shield is a thin piece of metal with a slit down the middle.

The mohel places the shield on the glans and pulls the foreskin through the slit. He slices off the foreskin and removes any remnants with his fingernails. The shield does not clamp the foreskin to the point of hemostasis (stopping blood flow). The shield is the mohel's most common instrument.[169]

2. Periah

With fingernails and scalpel, the mohel scrapes away any foreskin remains. Some mohels keep their fingernails sharpened to a point.

3. Metzitzah

A glass tube is used to suction up the blood. The mohel raises a cup of wine and says a prayer. He dribbles wine into the boy's mouth,[170] and applies a bandage below the glans at just the right tension to prevent further bleeding. He applies petroleum jelly to the glans and covers it with a swab.[171]

The mohel then says some blessings and names the child.

Non-orthodox Jewish ceremonies may not do all these same steps, but all do some cutting.

Witnessing a brit is quite different from having intellectual knowledge about it. At one brit I attended, the mother of the infant whispered to me, "This is barbaric!" But the ceremony went on.

Circ is emblazoned on the Jewish collective unconscious. As Jennifer Goodman, a Jewish physician, commented, "Circumcision became an emblem not just of faith, but of loyalty, courage, and the defiant fight for freedom against terrible oppression." Even nonpracticing Jews often religiously circumcise with a brit. One such man, who recognized his internal contradictions about it, published his thoughts in a Wall Street Journal article linked at the endnote.[172]

A case in Israel manifests the Jewish depth of attachment to circ. A father wanted to circumcise his son, but the mother refused, and they ended up arguing their case in court. The judge ruled that the boy would be circumcised, because it is essential for the soul, and for combating antisemitism.[173]

One common Jewish line of thinking is this: *We have survived for thousands of years, while other civilizations came and went. We must be doing something right! Why change a winning plan?*

A Hasidic man framed it this way: "From my father, going back to receiving the Torah on Mt. Sinai—that chain has not been broken. I'm frightened of losing that."[174] And another Hasidic man said, "Circ is of the utmost importance; it is our connection to God."[175] As a Jerusalem Post headline put it, "Jewish ritual is the secret to our survival."[176]

One mohel even believed, "My knife is so sharp that the child doesn't even feel the cutting." He then added, "The foreskin is a repulsive thing, that's why we remove it." Another mohel was philosophical about it, "I am an abuser. I circumcise because I am in covenant with God. Ultimately, God owns my morals, and my body."[177]

Miriam Pollack, a Jewish intactivist, noted how taboo it is to even discuss circ within the Jewish community.[178] Other Jews have made similar comments.[179] In a video linked at the endnote at the end of the sentence, one Jewish woman describes how her decision not to circumcise her son led to her being shunned by her synagogue and even her family.[180] I, too, have encountered strong resistance from some Jews when I discussed this book. "Some things are written in stone," scolded a friend.

Some Jews Question the Entire Brit

In the 1840s, a number of European Jewish leaders advocated abolishing circ, but nothing came of it.[181] In 1892, Reform Judaism did make a small concession by eliminating a circ requirement for adult converts to Judaism.[182]

Dr. Jennifer Goodman points out that babies may seem to be sleeping after the brit, but they are actually likely semicomatose due to what is called neurogenic shock.[183]

Rabbi Sherwin Wine, affiliated with the tiny Society for Humanistic Judaism, said, "There is no way of making a happy celebration out of the performance of bloody surgery."[184]

In 2011, anthropologist Leonard Glick estimated that one-sixth of American Jewish babies were being left intact,[185] and in Israel there is a growing movement to end circ too. A 2006 Israeli survey found that 5% of parents rejected circ for the following reasons: 2% were not Jewish, 2% objected to disfiguring the body, and 1% refrained because the act is painful. About one-third of parents preferred to circumcise because of either social pressure (17%), health (10%), or for the grandparents (2%).

Dr. Avshalom Zoossmann-Diskin, founder of Ben Shalem, an Israeli organization that fights circ, says he encountered only one harsh response over many years. It was in 1999, in connection with a petition that he submitted to the Israeli Supreme Court. It took a stand against circ, arguing that it violates Israel's Basic Law: Human Dignity and Freedom, and criminal law. The Israeli interior minister wrote in response, "The petitioner should be thrown out the window."[186]

In one Israeli survey of secular Jews, about half a million (7% of the population) either opposed or didn't care about circ.[187] "In Israel, circ opponents number in the tens of thousands," according to Ronit Tamir, founder of Kahal, a support group for parents who question circ.[188] She runs two Facebook groups—one for parents considering circ and the other for parents who choose not to circumcise. Each group has close to a thousand members.[189]

Alternatives to Brit Milah

In response to these evolving perspectives, non-surgical Jewish alternative ceremonies to Brit Milah have been proposed. They go by different names, but the most popular is Brit Shalom (covenant of peace), first coined by Rabbi Natan Segal in the early 1980s.[190]

As authors Rebecca Wald and Lisa Braver Moss said in their courageous groundbreaking book *Celebrating Brit Shalom*, "Couples today embrace natural, or positive parenting, including birth without unnecessary intervention, breast-feeding on demand, and close physical and emotional contact between care-giver and infant. Some feel circumcision is incompatible with those values."[191]

The book offers three possible ceremonies to replace circ. In each version, a pomegranate is cut, instead of a penis. "The pomegranate represents fertility and abundance," Wald said, "and it 'bleeds' when you cut it,"[192] reflecting the essence of the ceremony. The book contains sheet music, blessings, and other ideas. In 2021, the authors also launched Bruchim (a Hebrew amalgam of "blessed" and "welcome"), a group seeking to welcome non-circumcising Jews into the Jewish community.

When Braver Moss learned that half a dozen boys attending her synagogue preschool were intact, she was stunned. Even some rabbis were secretly aban-doning circ. In a revealing speech she gave, she disclosed policies that are keep-ing ceremonies like Brit Shalom hidden, and notes that some rabbis take the position "don't ask, don't tell." A link to a video of the speech is at the endnote.[193]

Her coauthor Wald maintains the Brit Shalom website www.beyondthebris.com, which has had hundreds of thousands of views since its inception in 2012. Rabbi Jerry Levy said that in recent years he has officiated at more Brit Shalom ceremonies than circs.[194]

Other names for alternative ceremonies include Brit B'li Milah (covenant without circ), Brit Chayim (covenant of life), and Brit Ben (covenant for a child).

Writer Jay Michaelson[195] has sensibly argued for a compromise alternative to the brit for traditional Jews not willing to give up circ. He suggests a minimal circumcision nick, as may have been done in biblical times. Professor Raphael Cohen-Almagor has suggested a weaker compromise: there should be a law that mohels train in anesthesia and be required to use it, but otherwise no changes.[196] Professor Hanoch Ben-Yami similarly recommends compulsory anesthesia and a ban on metzitzah.[197]

Other Jewish Voices against Circ

"In Judaism there is a law of *shmirat haguf* (protecting the body), so that body-piercing, tattooing, and amputation are all forbidden. Further, there is the Talmudic concept of compassion for all living creatures. If these were applied to eight-day-old babies, circumcision would be impossible."[198]—DR. JENNIFER GOODMAN

"I am Jewish and feel deeply harmed by circumcision. . . . I do not feel closer to Judaism because of it. . . . I wish one had nothing to do with the other."—BRIAN LEVITT, JEWISH INTACTIVIST, CO-FOUNDER OF JEWS FOR THE RIGHTS OF THE CHILD; TESTIMONY AT THE CALIFORNIA SENATE JUDICIARY COMMITTEE PUBLIC HEARING ON CIRCUMCISION.

Antisemitism, Philosemitism, and Circumcision

Criticizing circ places me uncomfortably close to people who oppose it solely because they hate Jews. For example, one vocal proponent of an initiative to ban circumcision in the city of San Francisco created horrific antisemitic cartoons as part of his presentation to the city council.[199]

Antisemitism is a worldwide plague, as it has been throughout history. I regularly read anti-Jewish sentiments online.

The Center for Digital Hate reported the following statistics regarding online platforms:

- Platforms failed to act on 81% of antisemitic posts.
- Facebook permits antisemitic groups to operate after exposure.
- Instagram, TikTok, and Twitter (now called X) allowed hashtags to be used for antisemitic content.
- YouTube has repeatedly failed to prevent antisemitic videos seen by millions. (And I have seen some of them.)
- TikTok removes just 5% of accounts that racially abuse Jewish users.[200]

The Qur'an (also spelled Koran), a book holy to two billion Muslims, has numerous vicious descriptions of Jews:

- liars (3:78, 2:10, 5:41)
- hypocrites (2:14, 2:44)
- evildoers (2:109 and 5:51)
- feel pain when others are happy (3:120)

- tricky thieves (4:161)
- prophet killers (2:61)
- merciless (2:74)
- extreme sinners (5:79)
- cowardly (59:13–14)
- miserly (4:53)
- apes and pigs (2:63–65, 5:59–60, 7:166)

Nor are these just ancient beliefs. One poll of the Muslim world showed that 74% harbor antisemitic beliefs.[201] I have read many similar polls over the years.

It is important to mention, that there are, of course, righteous Muslims who are not antisemitic. One such is Yasmine Mohammed, who wrote an eye-opening memoir about growing up Muslim in Egypt. Her aunt's anti-semitic obsession included warnings that Jews were somehow putting cancer into vegetables, and attacks on the output of anyone Jewish, including the theories of Albert Einstein, and the comedy of Jerry Seinfeld, on his TV show *Seinfeld*. Fortunately, Yasmine Mohammed is now a human rights activist.[202]

Note that none of the hatred I have listed is against Israelis—it pertains to all Jews, wherever they are found.

In *Jews Don't Count*, a brilliant book by David Baddiel, he shows how the West's view of Jews constantly shifts to place them in the worst possible light. Sometimes they're seen as a religious group, other times as an ethnic group or race. These days they don't count as a "real minority." He created the law "Schrödinger's Whites," in which Jews are White or non-White depending on the politics of the observer.[203]

After millennia of persecution, Jews see themselves as one of the most oppressed groups in history. Given this background, it's predictable that many Jews view attempts to ban circ as antisemitic attacks. For example, in 2012, a German court ruled that the circ of an infant male constituted "grievous bodily harm."[204] Although the ruling legally applied only to one doctor who circumcised a four-year-old Muslim boy, it "had a ripple effect, leading hospitals from Berlin to Zurich to suspend circumcision and emboldening a movement against the procedure that had previously gone largely unnoticed."[205]

German-Jewish communities decried the ruling. For example, Charlotte Knobloch, a former president of the Central Council of Jews in Germany, claimed pure antisemitism was behind anti-circ efforts.[206] Later, German lawmakers did a 180-degree turn and passed legislation guaranteeing the right of circ.[207]

In 2018, Iceland's government proposed banning circ. The Anti-Defamation League responded, "Should Iceland ban circumcision, making it impossible for Jews and Muslims to raise families in your country, we guarantee that neo-Nazis, white supremacists, and other extremists will celebrate Iceland."[208] The law didn't pass.

In 2020, in response to an anticircumcision conference, the director of international relations for the Simon Wiesenthal Center stated: "An attack on a fundamental ethic of Judaism can be construed as an assault on the Jewish people."[209]

It is understandable that Jews would see it that way, but alas this kind of attitude shuts down legitimate complaints about circ. Recognizing this, several prominent anticircumcision organizations and activists, both Jewish and gentile, including Attorneys For The Rights Of The Child, and Doctors Opposing Circumcision, issued a commendable joint policy statement entitled "Standing Against Antisemitism."[210]

But there is a flip side to these debates that could be called "philosemitism," meaning some gentiles are favorable towards Jews and therefore oppose attempts to ban circ. For example, according to John V. Geisheker, the executive director of Doctors Opposing Circumcision, many working doctors fear that they might be accused of antisemitism if they come out against circ.[211] And the United States Department of Health and Human Services stated, "Any attempt by a public agency to discourage non-medical circumcision could be misinterpreted as an attack on religious groups which practice it. It is not proper for government to adopt a policy that is directly or indirectly critical of a religious practice."[212]

It's also possible that some people are antisemitic at least in part *because* of circ. In some versions of antisemitic lore, circ is associated with the infamous blood libel, which refers to a centuries-old myth that Jews murder Christians to use their blood ritualistically, such as an ingredient of Passover matzah. Blood libels have frequently led to pogroms that decimated Jewish communities. This lie persists despite Jewish denials and repudiations by the Catholic Church and all civilized societies. I have read internet comments from people who believe in the blood libel.

Another terrible myth that circulates widely (and that I just read on the social media X platform) is that metzitzah is still being widely practiced by direct mouth sucking, whereas that is almost never the case anymore, as I explained above. The comments about it are outrageously vulgar and hateful.

Circ can still perplex even well-meaning people who don't believe these dastardly stories. Because of all of this, in my opinion, stopping Jewish circ would lead to less antisemitism.

Summary of Antisemitism and Circ
- Some antisemites will condemn circ purely out of hatred for Jews.
- Some Jews will see attacks on circ as antisemitic.
- Some gentiles who recognize that circ is harmful will nevertheless support it for fear of appearing antisemitic.
- Overall, circ increases antisemitism.

Jewish Identity and Change

The halacha firmly asserts that any child of a Jewish mother is considered Jewish regardless of beliefs or behaviors. So, circ is not a Jewish identity issue. Therefore, ending Jewish circ is possible without threatening Jewish peoplehood. And as Mordechai Kaplan, founder of the denomination of Conservative Judaism, famously put it, "Judaism is an evolving civilization."

As mentioned, the Orthodox Jewish core belief is the unaltered transmission of Jewish law since it was given on Mount Sinai. But various Jewish authorities have often been able to find work arounds to change things when they saw fit. As author Blu Greenberg put it, "Where there's a rabbinic will, there's a halachic way."

For example, Jews no longer perform animal sacrifices in the Temple, whose ceremonial details take up whole chapters in the Torah. There's no reason the Holy Temple couldn't be rebuilt, with sacrifices reinstituted, but there's no desire to do so, other than by a few fringe players. And slavery is now unthinkable, but it was a part of the circ verses and is pervasively mentioned throughout the Torah.

Here are some death-penalty offenses in the Torah, none of which are currently enforced as a capital crime:

- Striking or cursing one's parents (Exodus 21:15) (Exodus 21:17)
- Witchcraft (Exodus 22:17, Leviticus 20:15–16)
- Bestiality (Exodus 21:18 and 22:19; Leviticus 20:15–16)
- Worshiping other gods (Exodus 22:19 and 22:20; Deuteronomy 17:2–5)
- Doing forbidden activities on the Sabbath, for example, Numbers 15:32–36 describes how a man was stoned for gathering wood on the Sabbath
- Incest (Leviticus 20:11–12)
- Male-male sex (Leviticus 20:13)
- The daughter of a Cohen engaging in promiscuity (Leviticus 21:9)
- Blasphemy (Leviticus 24:14), for example, Leviticus 24:23 describes a stoning for blasphemy
- A nonvirgin woman marrying a man, as is found in the Deuteronomy 22:13–21 description of a woman being stoned
- A male having intercourse with an engaged virgin and her death being decreed if she could have cried out for help and did not (Deuteronomy 22:23–27)

———————

This is not to say that change is easy. In any group, even minor alterations of sacred rituals can be perceived as significant moral violations.[213]

Summary of Jewish Circ

In biblical times, circ was likely a custom among some Jews, possibly picked up from the Egyptians, whereby a bit of foreskin was removed.

Four major authors probably composed the Torah, with later emendations both accidental and intentional. Circ passages were added to the Torah by the last major author, P, over 700 years after the first author began the Torah.

In Greek and Roman times, as a backlash against attempts by Jews to reverse their circumcisions, Jewish authorities instituted periah and metzitzah to completely remove any foreskin. These radical modifications became obligatory, with Brit Milah configured as the most important ceremony in Judaism.

Metzitzah's direct application of the mouth to the penis was replaced in the 19th century with suction using a glass tube, but some Hasidic sects still perform the original practice. Jewish circ is a popular but likely declining practice among non-Orthodox Jews. Alternative ceremonies such as Brit Shalom, which involve no cutting, are on the rise. Antisemitism is a complex problem; more Jew hatred is generated by continuing to do circ.

MUSLIM CIRC

Muslims represent the largest group practicing circ. *Khitan* is the Arabic word for circ, also referred to as *tahera*, "purified."[214]

Unlike Jewish circ, Muslim circ is not a well-defined practice with clear protocols. The age at which circ is done, and the amount of foreskin removed, varies with regional, cultural, and individual preferences. For example, a Bangladeshi man told me that in his region Muslims did not even practice circ, whereas in Turkey 98% of Muslims do it.[215]

Overall, about 90% of Muslims circumcise.[216] On average, Muslim boys are circumcised at seven years old.[217] However, recently, some have been circumcising boys as young as two or three days old.[218] Circ is often done as a private ceremony, but there is a growing trend in Muslim communities to have a surgeon perform the act in a hospital.[219] It seems that anesthesia is not used for Muslim circ.

Why do Muslims circumcise? Abraham—the father of both Ishmael (founder of the Arab nation) and the Jewish patriarch Isaac—is revered by the Qur'an as "a guide for the people."[220] The Prophet Muhammad was ordered to follow the faith of Abraham (Qur'an 16:123), which is interpreted by some to include circ. The Hadiths are other Islamic holy texts that report Muhammad's deeds and sayings, and circ is mentioned in them, but not as a requirement. Also, a convert to Islam need not circumcise.

Special foreskin practices exist among some Muslim populations. In Iran, some place the excised foreskin on the circumcised boy's ankle to promote healing, and some wives add the foreskin to their husband's food as an aphrodisiac. In some Arab communities pregnant women swallow the foreskin to increase the odds of having a boy.[221]

Muslim circ is a festive ceremony, and the boy is typically dressed in a royal costume.

In another departure from Jewish practice, there is no Muslim equivalent to a mohel. Instead, a lay circ expert, or family member, often performs the procedure. Of course, when done in a hospital a doctor is the circumciser.

I spoke with a Muslim Turkish woman who observed the circumcision of her 9-year-old cousin at home. "He shrieked constantly, before, during, and after the circumcision. The entire family was traumatized." A *Vice* magazine reporter in Turkey wrote that there are many reports of circ complications in Turkey, from the trivial to the fatal.[222]

Surgeon Shiban Ahmed notes similar problems among Muslim circumcisions performed in England, and others report that poorly trained circumcisers and shoddy equipment cause problems.[223] The endnote links to a video of a seven-year-old Muslim boy who was justifiably outraged at his circumcision.[224] Sadly, the doctor and other men around him just laughed at him.

I could not find one Islamic procircumcision article except for a report by the World Health Organization that listed circ as one of five behaviors that Islamic men believe should be followed to be respectable. This list is from a sunnah, which is a teaching of Mohammed in the Hadiths. However, it is not clear if the reference is to male or female circ.[225] Also, many Muslim scholars have criticized the authenticity of sunnahs, finding problems of the types I described with the Torah.[226] For example, Mohammed Amin describes many internal contradictions within the Hadiths.[227] And Professor Mohammad Hashim Kamali also notes many instances where the Hadiths are contradicted by the Qur'an or by historical events.[228] To illustrate the depth of the skepticism, historian David Gollaher points out that even though there is a Hadith promoting Muslim female circumcision, it is considered of so little value that even advocates of the practice don't cite it.[229]

Some Islamic authorities, such as Ahmad Ibn Hanbal, Al-Nawawi, and Al-Tabari, have come out against circ.[230] Muslim preacher Ashraf Saad Mahmoud wrote that Muslim scholars disagree over whether circ is obligatory.[231] Professor Michael Rosen maintains it is not an Islamic requirement.[232]

There is also an Islamic fundamentalist movement called Quranism that reject Islamic traditions, such as circ, that aren't specifically named in the Quran.[233,234] Going a step further, Sami Aldeeb Abu-Sahlieh, at the Swiss Institute of Comparative Law, believes that circ even "violates the Koran." He cites these two Qur'anic passages:

"Our Lord, You did not create all this in vain" (3:191).
"[He] perfected everything He created" (32:7).[235]

Libyan judge Mustafa Kamal al-Mahdawi has argued that circ is purely a Jewish custom and has no place in Islam.[236] M. Cumhur Izgi,[237] Canadian

Muslim activist Arif Bhimji,[238] and Egyptian psychiatrist Nawal Al-Saadawi are other Muslim voices against circ.[239]

I conclude that most Muslim thinkers do not consider circ a necessity. Also, I found no documented instance of a Muslim being condemned because he wasn't circumcised. Kamel Elwazeir, president of the Islamic Society of Colorado Springs, notes that in Islamic communities, circ is considered a private matter, and no one inquires about your penile status.[240]

CHRISTIAN VIEWS OF CIRC

In the nascent years of Christianity, circ was abandoned, in part guided by the advice of the Apostle Paul.[241] Here are some New Testament quotes that reflect this:

> "Circumcision counts for nothing; its lack makes no difference. What matters is keeping God's commandments" (1 CORINTHIANS 7:18–19).

> "Watch out for workers of evil. Be on guard against those who mutilate" (PHILIPPIANS 3:2–4).

> "If you have yourselves circumcised, Christ will be of no use to you" (GALATIANS 5:2–6).

Despite this, some evangelical Christians,[242] and a few African Christian sects such as Coptic churches in Egypt, Ethiopia, and Eritrea, circumcise.[243]

Catholicism, in particular, is adamant about leaving boys intact. Circ is expressly forbidden on the grounds of respect for bodily integrity.[244] The Catechism of the Catholic Church paragraph number 2297 asserts, "Unless performed for strictly therapeutic medical reasons, amputations, mutilations, and sterilizations performed on innocent persons are against moral law."[245] The US Conference of Catholic Bishops adds: "All persons served by Catholic health care have the right and duty to protect and preserve their bodily and functional integrity. . . [except] to maintain the health or life of the person when no other morally permissible means is available."[246]

In 1442, the Catholic Church determined that circ was incompatible with salvation.[247] Pope Benedict XIV, Pope Pius XI, Pope Pius XII, and Pope Benedict XVI[248] have come out against circ. One Catholic bioethicist concluded, "It is unethical for Catholic health care institutions to allow neonatal male circumcision, except out of respect for religious practices of other faiths."[249] However, another Catholic website maintains that though the catechism proscribes mutilation, circ is not considered mutilation, and therefore should be permitted, but not mandated.[250]

Many American Catholics have chosen to circumcise. Of a number of Catholics I have discussed this with, none were cognizant of their church's stance. Many of them seemed to align with the ethos that "the only Catholic rule is to love another person," which was how Catholic scholar Dr. Gregory Popcak put it.[251] For more on Catholics speaking out against circ, see http://www.catholicsagainstcircumcision.org/.

OTHER RELIGIONS' VIEWS OF CIRC

Other major religions do not support circ,[252] but African or Australian Aboriginal circ practices may have a religious component.

———————

I've advanced a lot of arguments against religious circ, but I must acknowledge that our understanding of the world is always evolving, and sometimes ancient practices may have value, even if we don't understand their rationale. For example, in 2004, a cataclysmic tsunami claimed the lives of 230,000 people in southern Asia. However, among the indigenous people of the Andaman Islands, which were hit by 500-mile-per-hour waves, none were harmed. This remarkable outcome was attributed to their ancestral teachings, which impelled them to seek higher ground at the first sign of distress, though none could explain the custom's reason.[253]

SUMMARY OF RITUAL CIRC

Jewish circ started as a folk custom, possibly with a token penile nick and expanded to mandate complete foreskin amputation, based on manipulations of the Torah text and reactions to antisemitism. Muslim circ was never religiously mandated but is widely performed. No other major religions require circ.

"But, but—" I hear you say, "even if there aren't valid religious arguments for circ, isn't it medically beneficial?" In fact, every few years my local Jewish newspaper says it is.[254,255,256] Sample headline: "Circumcision is not only Jewish; it's good for you."

Is this true? Let's find out.

CHAPTER THREE

Medical Circumcision

or, Why I Ate Kellogg's Sugar
Frosted Flakes As a Child

THE HISTORY OF MEDICAL CIRC

Medical circ is the cutting of the foreskin purely for health reasons. As we have seen, circ disappeared from Christianity early on. Yet the largely Christian United States is the only country where most boys are medically circumcised, and that's due to a twisted historical process.

The path to circumcision began at the dawn of the Victorian era, with an obsession with the purported evils of masturbation, euphemistically called self-pollution. The 1716 pamphlet *Onania: Or, the Heinous Sin of Self-Pollution and All its Frightful Consequences, in Both Sexes, Considered with Spiritual and Physical Advice to Those who have Already Injured Themselves by This Abominable Practice*, exemplified this attitude.[257] Later, Dr. Benjamin Rush, a signer of the American Declaration of Independence in 1776, promoted the idea that masturbation was the cause of many illnesses.[258]

In 1835, Dr. Claude Francois Lallemand stated that boys masturbated because of irritation from "secretions" beneath the foreskin, which were likely just normal smegma. His view is symptomatic of a larger problem within Western medicine, with its preoccupation with disease, while deemphasizing well-being and physical pleasure. That's why Lallemand assumed a boy masturbated due to a medical condition—it couldn't just be because it felt good! He even invented a bogus medical condition called "spermatorrhea" (excessive ejaculations), which supposedly devastated the body. Thus, Lallemand transmogrified natural sexuality into a reprehensible and dangerous endeavor. But he had a solution: circ.[259]

Lallemand established medical principles that are still accepted today:

1. It is legitimate, and even necessary, to alter boys' genitals.
2. The boy's parents are the client, not the boy himself.[260]

Lallemand was French, but American business know-how took his ideas to the next level. Two of the greatest marketers in US history, Sylvester Graham, inventor of Graham crackers, and John Harvey Kellogg of cereal fame,[261] popularized the notion their bland, starchy foods could curb sexual desire and discourage masturbation.[262] According to Professor Howard Markel, Kellogg only promoted his cereals to improve digestion,[263] but it seems to me that Kellogg indicated that they also helped prevent masturbation.

Graham's imagination ran wild, "A masturbator becomes a confirmed degraded idiot, whose deeply sunken vacant glassy eyes, livid shriveled countenance, ulcerous toothless gums, fetid breath, feeble broken voice, emaciated dwarfish crooked body, bald—covered perhaps with suppurating blisters and running sores—denoting premature aging—a blighted body and ruined soul."[264]

It's possible that Graham was actually describing the symptoms of poisoning from lead or arsenic, found in some commonly used materials of that time, such as wallpaper and paint.[265]

Kellogg was the author of the 1888 bestseller *Treatment for Self-Abuse [masturbation] and its Effects*. Among the sadistic masturbation remedies he proposed were piercing the foreskin with wires to prevent erection and using carbolic acid to burn the clitoris. "Covering the organs with a cage has been practiced with entire success. Tying the hands is successful in some cases but will not always succeed." He also wrote, "Circ should be performed without anesthesia, so pain is associated with the habit we wish to eliminate."[266] (And if none of the above worked, Kellogg was a fan of eugenics.)

Kellogg finally decided that there were only two effective remedies for masturbation: Kellogg's cereals[267] and circ.[268] Kellogg was not consistent in his pronouncements and at one point said he was against routine circ[269] (though ostensibly it could still be used to "cure" masturbation.) Dr. Barbara Chubak believes that it was instead Dr. Lewis Sayre who promoted routine circ, around 1870.[270]

In 1895, British surgeon Sir Jonathan Hutchinson published the influential article "On Circumcision as a Preventative of Masturbation." Circ, he assured us, would prevent Satan from stealing a boy's soul via masturbation.[271]

These campaigns were so successful, that by 1910 the Encyclopedia Britannica described circumcision as a "surgical operation which is commonly prescribed for purely medical reasons," whereas before it had described it as a religious ritual.[272] Later, the US Marines deemed circ so vital that you couldn't enlist without it,[273] and in the 1930s, the US Boy Scout Manual cited the widely held belief that masturbation would make a boy weaker. The manual was only corrected in the late 1960s.[274] Even today, a common insult in the UK is calling a man a "wanker," (contemptible, literally a masturbator) a last remnant of Victorian thinking.

In the 1800s, the incentive for an American doctor to circumcise was great—he took the moral high ground and profited financially at the same time. So, many jumped on the self-abuse bandwagon and invented a myriad of rationalizations to justify circ, a trend that persists even today. Here is list of false claims from doctors about problems circ would ameliorate:

1845: "masturbation"—EDWARD DIXON

1855: "syphilis"—JONATHAN HUTCHINSON

1865: "epilepsy"—NATHANIEL HECKFORD

1870: "spinal paralysis"—LEWIS SAYRE (PRESIDENT OF THE AMERICAN MEDICAL ASSOCIATION!)

1873: "bedwetting"—JOSEPH BELL

1875: "scoliosis, paralysis of the bladder, clubfoot"—JOSEPH BELL

1879: "nocturnal emissions and abdominal neuralgia"—H. KANE

1881: "all eye problems"—MAXIMILLIAN LANDESBERG

1888: "masturbation, thus curing 31 different ailments"—JOHN HARVEY KELLOGG

1890: "blindness, deafness, and dumbness"—WILLIAM GENTRY[275]

1894: "Prevents African-Americans [he used a different word] from raping white women."[276] "Cures nearly 100 different conditions."[277]—PETER REMONDINO.

1900: "sensuality, syphilis and other disorders"—E. HARDING FREELAND[278]

1902: "priapism [persistent and painful erection of the penis], masturbation, and most functional nervous diseases of childhood"—L. EMMETT HOLT[279]

1914: "tuberculosis"—ABRAHAM WOLBARST[280]

1949: "prostate cancer, venereal disease, and cancer of the tongue"—EUGENE HAND[281]

1985: "urinary tract infections"—T. E. WISWELL[282]

2007: "HIV infection"—R. C. BAILY ET AL.[283]

More on these last two conditions, later.

In 1900, another factor led doctors to promote circ. Epidemiologists were trying to explain why Jews had lower rates of infectious diseases, such as syphilis and tuberculosis. One likely reason was that Jews in those days had little sexual contact with gentiles, who made up a substantial percentage of the population and had greater rates of these diseases. But some scientists wrongly concluded that the Jews' improved health was because of circ.[284]

In 1949, Dr. D. Gairdner massively added to the confusion by proclaiming that the foreskin should be fully retractable by age three.[285] In reality, the development of foreskin retraction is gradual,[286,287,288] with the average age of natural first foreskin retraction occurring at 10 years.[289] That's a fact that many doctors still don't know, as evidenced by attempts by too many of them to forcibly retract before the boy is ready (more on this later).[290] Unfortunately, Gairdner's findings gained widespread acceptance, which led to "false diagnoses of pathological phimosis and large numbers of medically unnecessary amputations of healthy foreskins."[291]

Finally, there is one more reason that US medical circ has become so popular: for-profit medicine. In that, circ joins a long list of medical procedures whose numbers are excessive. For example, one study concluded that as many as 1/3 of knee replacement surgeries are unnecessary.[292] Easy cash was also likely a prime motivator for yet another fashionable and uncalled for removal of one of my body parts—my tonsils.

Around birthing itself, circ is not the only questionable operation. Surgeries such as episiotomies (cutting the vagina to widen the opening) and Cesarean sections are also possibly overdone.[293] Further exploration of such birthing issues can be found at the website https://improvingbirth.org/.

All of these factors led to a peculiar intersection of square-peg-in-a-round-hole science, moral crusading, and greed, which set the stage for widespread acceptance of medical circ in the US.

But what exactly happens during medical circ?

MEDICAL CIRC PROCEDURE

In a typical medical circ, a boy less than one month old[294] is tightly strapped into a circumstraint.[295] Marilyn Milos, RN, attended one circumcision. She wrote, "[The baby had] a piercing scream when his foreskin was pinched and crushed as the doctor inserted an instrument between the foreskin and the glans, tearing the two structures apart. The baby started shaking his head back and forth—the only part of his body free to move—as the doctor used another clamp to crush the foreskin lengthwise, which he then cut. This made an opening large enough to insert a circumcision instrument. The baby gasped and choked, breathless from his shrill continuous screams. The doctor crushed the foreskin against the instrument and finally amputated it."[296]

And this was a normal circ with no complications. This experience was so jarring that Milos never participated in circ again, and in fact singlehandedly founded the modern American movement against circumcision.

The amount of foreskin removed in a medical circ is dependent on whatever agreement is done between the doctor and parents or guardian of the boy, but rarely is all of it removed, as in the Jewish tradition.

The most widely used circ instrument is the Gomco clamp, which crushes the foreskin with about 14,000 pounds (seven tons!) of force.[297] For context, that is about four times as strong as the highest bite force ever recorded, that of the Australian crocodile.[298] And as we'll see later, effective anesthesia is usually not used.

Does this sound like something you want to happen to your son? Intactivist Anthony Losquadro compares the use of circ clamps to someone slamming a car door shut on your finger, leaving it there for 15 minutes (to stop the bleeding), and then ripping off your fingernail.[299]

Let's discuss the pros and cons of medical circ.

POSSIBLE BENEFITS OF MEDICAL CIRC

Reduction in the Human Papillomavirus (HPV) Infection Rate

HPV is the most common sexually transmitted infection[300] and is usually transmitted by skin-to-skin genital contact.[301] In a minority of cases, HPV can be transmitted non-sexually, just by close contact.[302] Over 210 types of HPV have been identified, and about 15 types[303] (or 7%) may cause cervical cancer.[304,305] Cancer can appear years, or even decades, after an HPV infection. The types of HPV that cause genital warts differ from those that cause cancer.

HPV stands apart from all the other medical justifications because there is solid evidence that circ actually does reduce HPV infection rates in males and their female partners.[306,307] One study reported a 61% reduction and another 52%. The second study found the virus in various spots on the male genitalia, including parts of the foreskin, so it seems likely that the explains why circ helps—it removes locations where the virus hides out.

However, Gardasil 9 is a vaccine for HPV, and five studies have shown its tremendous efficacy.[308,309] For example, in 1 study, only 1 vaccinated woman in 6,016 developed diseases related to the dangerous forms of HPV.[310] The Centers for Disease Control and Prevention (CDC) recommends Gardasil 9 for all children at ages 11 to 12.[311] An mRNA-type HPV vaccine is also in the works.[312]

Also, since the 1950s, cervical cancer cases and deaths have dropped sharply, primarily because of the Papanicolaou (Pap) screening test. Moreover, the newer HPV test is superior to the Pap test for detecting early signs of cervical cancer, which should further reduce cancer cases, and provide less incentive to circumcise.[313]

Given the availability of a vaccine, the drop in the cancer rate, and the possibility of non-sexual HPV transmission, why take the drastic preventive measure of slicing off a body part?

Reduction in HIV/AIDS Rate

Studies done between 2005 and 2007 claimed that circ reduced rates of HIV acquisition in males during sexual intercourse with HIV-positive women by a fantastic 60%. The studies were done in Kenya,[314] South Africa,[315] and Uganda.[316] But the results do not hold up to scrutiny.

First, some perspective. The percentages represent a relative risk reduction. For example, in the South African study, the rate of HIV acquisition in circumcised males was 0.85%, and that in the intact group was 2.1%. The *relative* difference was 60%, but the absolute difference was only

2.1% − .85% = 1.25%.

So, in reality, proponents are proposing circumcising all males for a small 1.25% absolute drop in HIV infection rates.

———————

There were many problems with the studies, which had a circ group and a non-circ control group:

- The circ group received more condoms and safe sex counseling and were more inclined to use the condoms. This skewed the results toward making the circ group look safer than it was.[317]
- The circ group abstained from sex for at least six weeks after circ, but the control group did not; however, the statistics didn't account for this fact, which also made the circ group seem safer.
- A substantial number of participants contracted HIV from nonsexual sources: 23 of 69 (33%) infections in the South African study and 16 of 67 (24%) in the Ugandan study. That means for a significant number of cases, the issue of circ had nothing to do with HIV acquisition.[318]
- Van Howe noted that applying the statistical "Cochran risk of bias tool 2.0," these trials are at considerable risk for statistical bias and lacked robustness.[319] Specifically, if just 1 or 2 patients more per 1000 had *not* benefited from circ, it would have nullified the studies' statistical significance.
- All three studies ended early, which exaggerates the benefit of circ,[320] because when randomized controlled trials are stopped early for benefit, the treatment effects are exaggerated.
- Circ was not beneficial for women having sex with HIV-positive men,[321,322] and it increased women's HIV risk by the same margin that it is claimed to reduce men's risk.[323] This means that the net effect of on an entire population would be zero. This last study was ended early because too many women were becoming infected through their partners' recent circ wounds. If this effect occurred in a clinical trial setting with optimal counseling, it would likely be much worse in the real world.

———————

An African circ campaign began in earnest in March 2007, when the World Health Organization (WHO) and the Joint United Nations Programme on HIV/AIDS (UNAIDS) convened a consortium of researchers and public health experts to discuss these studies. Numerous participants reported that anticircumcision voices were stifled. For example, Gary Dowsett, the deputy director of the Australian Research Centre in Sex, Health and Society, characterized the three days' extended discussions as a one-sided presentation of circ's benefits that trampled dissent.

To be fair, there was an atmosphere of desperation in 2007 because AIDS was devastating Africa, and there was no treatment.[324] However, AIDS is no longer the death sentence that it once was. With consistent antiretroviral therapy, HIV-infected people can expect a near-normal lifespan.

In 2022, a statistical analysis of African HIV rates found that circ did not reduce HIV rates. As of this writing in 2024, it's been 17 years since these three African studies were done, and they haven't been replicated.

A meta-analysis (an evaluation of all the studies on this topic) determined that HIV prevention was not a reason to circumcise.[325] Based on all these findings, various authors have concluded that there is no evidence that circ reduces HIV transmission.[326,327,328,329,330]

John Erickson supplies a dose of common sense against circ for HIV prevention by noting that the keratinized penis of a circumcised man would be more likely to cause vaginal abrasions through which HIV can enter.[331]

Finally, consider this: Even if the studies were true, does it make sense to amputate an infant's valuable erogenous tissue because he'll have a 1.25% less chance of getting a non-fatal disease many years into the future?

Other HIV and Circ Studies

The largest study to date has been a 2021 study of a colossal 570,000 Canadian males, which found that circ was not related to the rate of HIV acquisition.[332] The same applied to a study of Danish males.[333]

———————

One technical note: When I cite medical articles, I may only use the author's last name, as is common practice in medical literature.

Kenyon et al. demonstrated that the large variation in HIV prevalence in different ethnic groups is explained not only by the prevalence of circ but also by sexual behavior.[334] For example the Luo (an African ethnic group) had high rates of HIV, with possibly contributions from more HIV testing (which discovered it more), and more promiscuous sex.

A study in India that was correlational and observational found that circ reduced HIV rates in men, but also noted, in contradistinction, that circ wasn't protective for Hindu men, who made up 34% of the sample. This implies that there's another factor in HIV acquisition which is not being accounted for.[335] The study also didn't measure whether HIV was acquired from infected needles, which accounts for 7% of US HIV cases.[336] All of this confusion makes it difficult to draw any conclusions from this study.

Another HIV study done in Kenya of truckers (different from the Kenyan study mentioned above) correlated HIV with intactness.[337] As anthropologist Leonard Glick pointed out, these men commonly had sex with HIV-infected sex workers, which is a more likely explanation for high HIV levels than being intact.[338]

Two studies of male-to-male sex showed, that regarding HIV transmission, there was "no overall protective benefit" from circ.[339,340]

In 2023, a small Chinese study reported at a conference claimed that circ reduced rates of HIV acquired from male-to-male sex. However, the study has not been published or peer reviewed, and it did not control well for what they refer to as "pre-exposure prophylaxis therapy," in other words, safe sex practices.[341]

Finally, a study in Uganda of HIV transmission in monogamous, heterosexual couples in which only one partner was already infected found that the circumcision status of the male partner was not a significant factor.[342]

––––––––––

The pro-circ 2012 UNAIDS report[343] cites on the very first page the three flawed African studies I cited at the beginning of this section. The same UN committee reported in 2019 of "remarkable progress in the scale up of voluntary medical male circ."[344] However, the committee was only commenting on the success of getting circ done and did not report any actual results regarding HIV. They only *assumed,* based on their mathematical models, that this had saved lives.

The WHO and UNICEF issued a report on violations of children's rights, which mentioned female circumcision but failed to mention male circ.[345] And in other WHO reports, the authors described only the negative effects of female circ, and only the positive effects of male circ.[346,347]

Based on these flawed AIDS studies, there have been massive circ campaigns in Africa. How did they fare?

Results of African Mass Medical Circ

Between 2008 and 2018, 23 million males underwent circ in 14 African countries.[348] A South African study found that these men had a *higher* prevalence of HIV than intact men. The authors offered a possible explanation: circumcised men wrongly concluded that they could engage in risky sex behaviors.[349] A Dutch study, discussed in more detail later, showed the same thing. Another possible reason for these results may be that circumcised men have more trouble attaining sexual satisfaction, such as in Botswana, where circ was correlated with promiscuity and transactional sex.[350]

There are six countries in Africa where men tend to be *more* HIV positive if they've been circumcised: Cameroon, Ghana, Lesotho, Malawi, Rwanda, and the Kingdom of Eswatini (formerly called Swaziland).[351] No countries' populations had lower HIV rates if they were circumcised.

Another South African study did find a greater rate of syphilis in intact men. However, the circumcised group used condoms more (perhaps because they were more concerned about STIs, which is why they got circumcised to start with), so of course they had less syphilis.[352] This is just one more example of the problems with real-world medical testing.

A 2021 study of 8 countries in sub-Saharan Africa showed that for men 15 to 59 years old, circumcised males had a 57% *greater* incidence of HIV. The circ group had a 1.4% incidence rate, versus 0.89% in the non-circ group.[353]

Swaziland set out to circumcise 80% of adult men in 2011, but only about 6% underwent the procedure. Interviews demonstrated that most Swaziland men were apparently wiser than their American counterparts. The Swaziland resisters correctly believed that circ resulted in reduced penis sensitivity and sexual pleasure and increased possible post-operative complications.[354]

A 2023 study of how circ fared in five African countries did show a small reduction in rates of HIV and syphilis.[355] However, this was a retrospective correlational study, and as the study admits, cannot establish cause and effect. It seems probable that men concerned enough about sexual risks to get circumcised would take other safe sex precautions too, so this study proves nothing.

Another problem with African circ is the risk. For example, of 443 males circumcised traditionally (at home) in Kenya, 35% experienced an adverse event compared with 18% of men who were circumcised in a medical facility. Bleeding and infection were the most cited adverse effects, with excessive pain, lacerations, torsion, and erectile dysfunction also reported.[356] The World Health

Organization noted that the rate of death and penile amputations from African tribal circ is "alarmingly high."

As a result of the problems with these circ campaigns, African anticircumcision organizations have been set up, including The VMMC (Voluntary Medical Male Circumcision) Experience Project[357] and Intact Kenya.[358]

Other ways to prevent AIDS are being considered. First, there is a proposed preventive drug regimen for AIDS. A *Journal of the American Medical Association* article recommended that people at high risk for HIV infection should prophylactically take certain HIV drugs. One brand—a two-medication combo pill named Truvada—is approved for preventive use in the US.[359]

Second, HIV vaccines are in development at Moderna Therapeutics and other companies. An initial vaccine was 30% effective but rejected as insufficiently protective. A vaccine would benefit all genders, whereas, at best, as I mentioned, circ only reduces HIV rates for men.[360] Two studies concluded that there will eventually be an approved vaccine.[361,362] In June 2024, Gilead Sciences' lenacapavir drug was shown to prevent a miraculous 100% of HIV cases when taken only twice a year.[363] As of this writing, it has just passed Phase 3 trials, and is nearly certain to obtain FDA approval.

Third, Excision BioTherapeutics is working on CRISPR gene-editing approaches to preventing AIDS.[364]

HIV Summary

There is insufficient evidence to support circumcising men to reduce the incidence of AIDS. Circ may slightly reduce HIV transmission from females to males, but it increases transmission in the opposite direction, leading to no net benefit for a population. Mass circ campaigns have actually increased HIV prevalence. Better solutions to combating HIV would be the use of vaccines, condoms, and, for high-risk populations, preventive drugs like lenacapavir.

Reduction of Sexually Transmitted Infections other than HIV

There is a myth that circ reduces sexually transmitted infections (STIs) (also called sexually transmitted diseases, or STDs). But a 1987 study found that circ increased the incidence of an STI known as nongonococcal urethritis (NGU).[365] Other studies found that there was no correlation between circ status and either

NGU or gonorrhea,[366] and no relationship between circ and herpes simplex virus type 2 infection.[367] It is possible that the lysozyme in the foreskin protects against STIs. The word lysozyme literally means "dissolves enzymes" and lysozymes are both antibacterial and antiviral.

In 2021, a massive, 30-year study of Danish males reported that circ was associated with *higher* STI rates overall, particularly for anogenital warts and syphilis.[368] This may be explained by another Dutch study that reported that immigrant (mostly circumcised) males have a greater tendency to engage in risky sexual behavior with prostitutes compared with native Dutch (mostly intact) males.[369] Another possible cause is that circumcised men, who have much less sensitivity than intact men, are significantly less likely to use condoms,[370,371] thus increasing their chances of getting an STI.

In general, Europe, with its low rate of circ, has significantly less STIs than the US. See a link to a graph of this at this endnote.[372]

Ethical Considerations of Doing Circ to Prevent STIs

STIs usually occur only after sexual maturity. If prevention of STIs is being used as a circ rationale, then shouldn't it be postponed until boys are old enough to decide for themselves?

Reduction of Penile Cancer Rate

In 1932, Wolbarst proposed that having a foreskin increases penile cancer risk. Even if that were true, penile cancer is extremely rare, occurring in about one man in 166,000 (or 6/1,000,000).[373] However, even according to pro-circ activist Brian Morris, approximately 33% of penile cancers are caused by HPV, leaving 67% due to other conditions.[374] So for men who get the Gardasil 9 vaccine, which virtually eliminates their HPV risk, the odds of getting penile cancer decrease to an extremely small

0.67(6) per 1,000,000 = 4 per 1,000,000

or

1 in 248,756 men.

In addition, penile cancer is primarily a disease of later years—the average age of diagnosis is 68 years.[375] But since some infants who are preventively "treated" for penile cancer by circ may not even live to old age, the actual odds of the circumcised infant (who later gets the HPV vaccine) getting penile cancer in later life are going to be less than 1 in 248,756. Contrast this with the odds of being hit by lightning over a lifetime: 1 in 15,300.[376] In other words, a man vaccinated with Gardasil 9 is 16 times more likely to be hit by lightning than to get penile cancer.

Another consideration is that penile cancer is not a death sentence; it has a good survival rate.[377] Finally, there are far more deaths from circ itself than there are from penile cancer, and not only that, circ raises the chance of other types of cancers, which I will show later. Taking all of the above into account, it makes no sense to circumcise a boy to prevent penile cancer.

Reduction in Urinary Tract Infection Rate

Urinary tract infection (UTI) can affect the kidneys, ureters, bladder, or urethra. The rate of UTI in infant boys is 1% to 2%,[378] and the standard treatment is 7 to 14 days of antibiotics.[379] More serious complications occur in only 1 in 5,236 cases.[380]

In 1985, T. E. Wiswell et al. published a study proposing that circ reduces the incidence of UTIs.[381] The AAP called the study flawed[382] and added that there are no reported cases of UTI in intact male infants without urinary birth defects.

Other studies have contradicted Wiswell et al. as well.[383,384] However, a meta-analysis in 2024 did find that circ reduced the risk of UTIs. But the meta-analysis was extremely biased toward being procirc, as shown by its selectively ignoring anticirc studies. It also admitted that UTIs are generally a minor problem and "long-term sequelae from UTI are unlikely if the urinary tract is normal."[385]

Amir et al. maintained that circ actually increases the risk of UTIs.[386] One study found that circumcised boys are 21 times more likely to develop urinary tract problems.[387] And circ leaves the meatus (peehole) open for bacteria to invade the urinary tract, since it doesn't have its protective foreskin cover.[388]

Two studies pointed out that even if circ reduced the incidence of UTIs, for every case it prevents, it creates two cases of hemorrhage or infection.[389,390]

Finally, three studies have found that UTIs seem to occur more frequently after Jewish ritual circ than medical circ.[391,392,393] This might be because typical brit settings may not be as sterile as a hospital.

Related to UTI is urinary retention, which means difficult or even impossible urination. It is a common complication of circ.[394] It can cause abdominal distension[395] and even kidney failure.[396]

From all the above, it seems that circ is not worth doing to prevent UTIs.

Hygiene

Just as personal hygiene routines like tooth brushing are essential, intact males need to clean their foreskin once it becomes retractable.

Some have proposed that circ makes hygiene less time consuming. However, the foreskin just needs to be rinsed periodically, which amounts to just a few seconds a day of care. Unfortunately, some areas of the world have limited amounts of water. Even so, according to Dr. M. Hakim, who lives in such an area, even infrequent rinsing is sufficient to maintain the foreskin.[397] So, hygiene is not a valid reason to circumcise.

Conformity of Appearance

A survey highlighted the significance of appearance conformity, revealing that the top reason parents chose circumcision was to ensure the baby resembled his father or others in his community.[398] However, no study has demonstrated any bad effects for a boy whose penis appears unlike those of others around him.[399]

One woman I interviewed said, "My son, born in 1971, was not circumcised, at a time when most boys were. He never experienced any mocking." Another woman told me a similar story.

Treatment of Phimosis

Phimosis is the inability to completely retract the foreskin and expose the glans. Up to this point I have discussed the dubious benefits of routine circ of a healthy penis. The treatment of phimosis falls in a different category: circ to treat a condition. However, even here, circ is usually unnecessary.

Infant boys' foreskins don't retract, and they should be left that way;[400] two studies found that only 36% of physicians knew this.[401] Boys will naturally retract their foreskin when it is ready to happen, typically as they approach adolescence. Trying it before that is painful and could cause long-term damage.[402]

One US study found that around 1 in 200 intact boys will develop a medical condition (usually phimosis) necessitating circ,[403] and a similar rate was found in Denmark.[404] However, a British study concluded that only 1 boy in 2500 had true phimosis (but 8 times that number were being treated for it).[405] And The Finnish Board of Health estimates Finland's phimosis rate at 0.023%—a tiny 1 in 50,000 cases.[406] Why the discrepancy? It's likely due to a lack of education among US physicians, so probably the 1 in 200 US phimosis rate actually includes a lot of misdiagnosed healthy boys who were just not old enough for retraction to occur naturally. As Bollinger noted, most North American doctors do not understand proper foreskin dynamics.[407] As recently as 1997, many physicians were still proposing improper and damaging forced retraction of newborns.[408] And one survey showed that many teenage boys didn't even know their foreskin could retract.[409] So there is an education problem with both doctors and patients.

For true phimosis, conservative treatments other than circ usually work. Varghese and Mathew believe only 4% of phimosis cases require surgery.[410] The US study cited above reported that 0.5% of boys have phimosis that needs circ. If Varghese and Mathew are right, that means that only 4% of that 0.5%, or a miniscule 0.02% (1 in 5,000) truly needed surgery.

Further, a meta-analysis of randomized controlled trials of phimosis studies plus two other studies all concluded that phimosis should be treated with topical steroid cream, which is more effective and less painful and costly than circ. Steroid cream is the most common non-surgical intervention and has a high success rate, with the added benefit of maintaining the penis's appearance.[411,412,413] If the patient is an adult, these treatment decisions should be made by him.[414]

A newer non-surgical phimosis treatment uses a device called PhimoStop which progressively stretches the foreskin's cells over time. It boasts an 81% success rate.[415] A similar device, called the Novoglan Foreskin Extender Treatment, also had a positive study,[416] but the manufacturer sponsored it, so it has to be replicated to be trusted.

Even more stubborn cases don't require circ either. For example, preputioplasty, also known as "limited dorsal slit with transverse closure," is surgery to widen a narrow foreskin that cannot comfortably be drawn back off the glans during erection. It can be performed with a local anesthetic in a doctor's office and rapidly heals with no significant change in appearance. One study concluded that preputioplasty is a valid option in the treatment of extreme phimosis.[417]

Even if circ is decided upon, only a partial circ is necessary to alleviate the problem. There are no documented cases of phimosis necessitating complete foreskin removal.

Also, if phimosis is treated with circ, it may make things worse. There's one case of circ leading to such chronic pain that the patient committed suicide.[418] We don't know the prevalence of long-term pain from circ.

Finally, some adult men have foreskins that do not retract, but it's not a problem if it doesn't interfere with sexual intercourse, and as far as hygiene, urination cleans the inside of the foreskin.

Another type of phimosis is called "secondary phimosis," and it occurs when an adhesion of remaining postcircumcision foreskin interferes with retraction. So instead of circ treating phimosis, it can actually cause it. We don't know its prevalence but from May 2015 to June 2019, 134 boys were treated for circ-caused phimosis at just one outpatient clinic. It is most commonly seen after Plastibell circ (a common circ device that will be discussed in Chapter 8).[419]

Treatment of Lichen Sclerosus

Another condition that could possibly be treated with circ is lichen sclerosus, also known as balanitis xerotica obliterans (BXO), an autoimmune inflammatory skin disease, commonly appearing as whitish patches on the genitals. It affects about .4% of males and can cause significant discomfort.[420,421]

The gold-standard treatment is three months of high potency topical steroids. Second-line pharmaceutical treatments include two drug types: topical calcineurin inhibitors (immunosuppressants) and imiquimod (an immune response modifier). In the rare case that none of these work, a minimal cutting can be tried.[422]

Mervyn Lander, a pediatric surgeon with 27 years of experience, states that foreskin BXO is the only medical reason to circumcise. He adds that circ for a healthy baby persists due to mindless inertia of the medical system.[423]

A new treatment for BXO is autologous platelet-rich plasma (PRP). This therapy uses injections of a patient's own platelets to promote healing. In one study, PRP was 100% successful in treating BXO of patients who had not responded to all other therapies.[424] The study sample size of five was too small to be reliable, but hopefully it will be replicated with more subjects. PRP is a treatment in growing use in medicine for a variety of conditions (I received it for a torn tendon).

Marilyn Milos believes that some cases of BXO are actually yeast overgrowth that can be treated with bacterial replacement therapy via probiotics.[425]

Mistaken Intact Attacks

Some health professionals complain about problems with patients with intact penises. I have read these comments on the social media platform X. But it is likely that these issue are caused by inadequate hygiene or too-early attempts at retraction. One pediatrician I spoke with evaluated an intact boy whose parents unfortunately tried to retract his foreskin in infancy, which led to scar tissue that eventually became infected. I wonder how many infections are due to too-early retraction, which can tear tissue and allow pathogens to take hold.

Another largely preventable problem with staying intact is foreskin yeast infections. Often these come when soap is used to clean under the foreskin, which is always a mistake. The soap strips natural emollients from the mucosal surface and alters the pH, allowing the yeast *candida albicans* to grow. For treatment options, see the link at this endnote.[426]

Summary of Possible Benefits of Circ

The only significant medical benefit of routine circumcision is to reduce transmission of HPV; however, an effective HPV vaccine is a much better solution.

There are two rare medical conditions that circ may benefit: phimosis and BXO, both of which usually have better treatments than circ. Even if circ is done for these conditions, it is usually only necessary to remove a minimal amount of foreskin. The need for medical circ is very rare, and in cultures such as Finland where it is not the norm, only one boy in 50,000 is circumcised.[427]

HARMS FROM CIRC

Now that we've covered circumcision's alleged benefits, let's look at the much longer list of problems that it might generate.

Pain

Mohel Henry Romberg writes, "When I officiate at a bris, I try to make it not only a wonderful *simcha* (joyous occasion) for all concerned but also a learning experience."[428] Really? Circ is certainly not joyous for the infant!

Academia has recognized infant pain for a long time. As early as 1925, a study noted that infants react to pin pricks,[429] and a notable 1987 Harvard study delineated the anatomical pathways and mechanisms for pain perception in infants.[430]

Pain is difficult to measure in a newborn who can't self-report, but magnetic resonance imaging (MRI) brain scans demonstrate that babies experience pain just like adults or perhaps more so. They also have a lower pain threshold.[431]

In addition to MRIs, checklist scales can evaluate infant pain[432] by measuring external manifestations of pain, such as shrieking, crying, and distorted facial features. Other measures are internal: heart rate, levels of cortisol (the stress hormone), respiratory rate, and brainwave activity.

All these measures yield the same result: Circ is excruciating,[433] not only during the procedure but also in the days that follow, marked by "severe and persistent pain."[434] Ryan calls it "the most painful procedure in neonatal medicine."[435] Williamson notes, "This level of pain would not be tolerated by older patients."[436] One study noted that circ is so painful that it is the model for newborn pain.[437]

Pediatrician Paul Fleiss considered infants' cortisol levels and heart rates during circ to be "consistent with torture."[438] And the pain can be further exacerbated after surgery as acidic urine might burn the circ wound. Nurses report that circumcised boys appear distant and don't behave normally.[439]

A 1997 study tested various types of anesthesia for infant circ. Control group babies received no anesthesia, but they were in such agony that some began choking, and one even had a seizure. How could it be otherwise? The foreskin evolved to promote sensation, not to resist being cut. The study was stopped.[440]

But pain numbers don't capture the whole experience. For one thing, pain is subjective; for example, when an adult undergoes a painful procedure, holding the hand of a loved one reduces the pain level.[441] In medical circ, the baby is typically strapped down, and just being restrained is distressing to newborns.[442] The helplessness makes it even more unbearable.[443] Psychologist Justin Call characterizes infants' crying from circ as abnormal and such a sign of distress that the babies sometimes lapse into a coma.[444] General anesthesia usually cannot be used on a newborn, and even when using the best local anesthesia techniques, circ pain is still significant.[445]

Maybe you're thinking . . . OK, it's painful, but infants don't remember, so there are no long-term consequences. But David Chamberlain, a child psychologist, relates how his two-year-old granddaughter remembered being hurt by a needle stick used to take a blood sample, when she was a newborn.[446] And a landmark study conducted six months after circumcision, reported that circ infants showed greater response to vaccination pain than intact infants.[447] Nobody has measured the pain response beyond six months—it could last a lifetime. Another study showed that infant pain causes significant consequences to all these systems: central nervous, endocrine, and immune.[448] In line with this, Fitzgerald and Beggs believe extreme pain in infancy "can lead to prolonged alterations in pain pathways that can last into adult life."[449] A recent study elucidated how the brain is changed by trauma;[450] these negative experiences are likely encoded in the amygdala.[451]

Anesthesia for Circ

In a traditional brit, the boy gets some drops of wine, or sugar water, which are feel-good efforts that do not provide any anesthesia[452] and are administered *after* the cutting. A mohel has no license to use pharmaceutical anesthesia unless he is also a physician.

"Doing things in sensitive parts of the body without anesthesia is cruel,"[453] said Sylvia Fine, MD. And physicians Rabinowitz and Hulbert call circ without anesthesia "barbaric."[454]

When circ is done in a hospital, EMLA cream—a mixture of lidocaine 2.5% and prilocaine 2.5%—is sometimes used.[455] However, it is a mild anesthetic that is intended, according to the manufacturer, "to temporarily numb the surface of skin prior to procedures such as needle insertion and minor skin surgery. It should not be applied *to the genitals of children* (emphasis mine)." So the manufacturer of the cream warns directly that it should not be used for circ because it's for surface numbing, not amputation.[456]

The second type of common anesthesia is a dorsal penile block (often a lidocaine injection at the base of the penis). In this case, using EMLA cream to dull the pain of the needle makes sense.

———————

Other types of anesthesia for circ that have been experimented with but are not widely adopted include the following:

- Recent studies used ketamine as an anesthetic, with favorable results.[457,458,459]
- Studies showed improved results when using an ultrasound-guided injection of a penile block (The ultrasound makes it easier to find the precise location for insertion of the needle.).[460,461]
- Injections near the anus (known as a perianal block) or near the tailbone (a caudal block) have been attempted.[462]
- Another recent experimental technique was used for Muslim circ of children. A Google virtual reality device diverted attention from the procedure by creating a familiar environment. It was useful in reducing the anxiety level of children during circ.[463] A more

sophisticated virtual reality device is called a SmileyScope.[464] Studies have shown that it reduces pain during procedures by up to 60% and is FDA-approved for treatment of children (but it wouldn't work for infants).[465]

The best circ anesthesia procedure (although still only partially effective) would use a penile block injection preceded by EMLA cream.[466] The EMLA cream must be applied at least 15 minutes before the block (time estimates vary widely), and the block takes 30 minutes to take effect, so that's a total of 45 minutes of preparation before circ. Therefore, it's predictable that, based on numerous anecdotes, most circ surgeons don't bother with anesthesia at all.[467,468,469,470,471,472] This was confirmed by a survey that found that only 38% of physicians used the penile nerve block.[473] This figure was based on self-report, so the true percentage was probably lower. When questioned why they didn't use the block, respondents cited "concern over adverse drug effects" (54%) followed by "procedure does not warrant anesthesia" (44%) as the most frequent explanations. None reported the obvious: Time is money. And according to at least one surgeon, those who use EMLA cream don't even wait the required time for it to set in, so it's ineffective.[474]

Even minimal palliative care might not be done. A circumcision nurse commented, "One doctor cautioned us against saying 'poor baby' and stroking him, which we do with anything else that hurts a baby, such as inoculating him."[475]

The stance of the prestigious *New England Journal of Medicine's* is that inadequate pain control is unethical.[476] And according to widely accepted ethical guidelines,[477] surgery cannot even be performed on *animals* without adequate anesthesia.[478] There are no such protections for human infants.[479] Circ somehow seems always to slip through the cracks.

As mentioned before, even with the best anesthesia, no way has been found to make it pain free.[480,481] Also, the anesthesia wears off in hours, but the pain lasts about 12 days."[482]

At a brit, Reform and Conservative mohels tend to use anesthetic more than Orthodox mohels, although it is likely they're only using the nearly useless EMLA cream. No Jewish denomination mandates the use of an anesthetic, but none objects to it either.[483]

How did this neglect of pain happen? It began when the CDC adopted the American Academy of Pediatrics' circumcision policy, which further gave weight to it. In that report, the CDC offered misleading pain guidance for circ that many physicians rely on as a standard of practice. The CDC barely mentions pain in their circ report,[484] because they cite a study by Banieghbal stating that only 7% of neonates experienced significant pain from circ.[485] But this is misleading. First, the CDC cherry-picked this study, ignoring all the other damning pain studies I cited above. Second, the Banieghbal study is of infants who received penile block anesthesia during circ, which is not usually the case. Moreover, the CDC ignored the pain of the injection itself.[486,487]

An American Academy of Pediatrics task force that investigated general infant pain from all types of procedures concluded that pain can be profound and may lead to long-lasting pain sensitivity. Because of this, a new AAP policy statement recommends reducing the severity and frequency of painful surgeries as much as possible. However, circ wasn't mentioned in that policy statement.[488]

In general, pain in medicine often doesn't receive the attention it deserves. Dr. Ross Zbar discovered this the hard way when he underwent an agonizing tracheostomy (the insertion of a tube into the windpipe), which he described in his book *Floating Feathers: A Doctor's Harrowing Experience as a Patient Within Conventional Medicine—and an Impassioned Call for the Future of Care in America*. This technique is so outmoded that it was first described during the Roman Republic. Less painful techniques have been invented but are not widely used, which Dr. Zbar found baffling.[489]

Trauma

Psychiatrist Richard Schwartzman postulates that the earlier a trauma takes place, the more detrimental it is,[490] with trauma during the first couple of months of life being the most damaging of all.[491]

For example, a study done almost 70 years ago showed that among children undergoing surgery for various conditions, there was a strong association between the age of the child at the time of the operation and the frequency and severity of emotional sequelae (secondary results), and 42% of children less than three years old at the time of operation had psychological problems, compared with only 10% among older children who had surgeries.[492] Victoria and Murphy argue that early life trauma even affects immune function.[493]

Specific trauma findings in regard to circ are as follows:

- A groundbreaking study showed that men circumcised in child-hood had, as adults, lower attachment security (feeling safe in a relationship) and emotional stability, and higher perceived stress and sensation-seeking behaviors compared with intact men.[494] This is ironic, because one of the reasons put forth for circ was that it combats lust.

- Among Filipino preadolescent and adolescent boys, almost 70% of the boys subjected to ritual circ (tuli, described above) and 51% of those who had medical circ had post-traumatic stress disorder (PTSD).[495,496] As a point of comparison, the PTSD rate of Iraq war veterans is 20%.[497]

- Boys aged four to seven who underwent circ often perceived the procedure as damaging and mutilating and commonly experienced feelings of inadequacy and helplessness, leading to withdrawal.[498] Dan Bollinger reported that circumcised boys were more likely to undergo adverse childhood experiences such as abuse, violence, and neglect.[499] He hypothesizes that this is because the trauma of circ could be as damaging as growing up in types of dysfunctional house-holds, such as those marred by violence or alcoholism.

- One month after circ, an MRI of an infant showed significant evi-dence of trauma in the amygdala, and frontal and temporal lobes of the brain.[500]

- Developmental neuropsychologist James Prescott maintains that circ affects brain development, and its pain, "limits subsequent experi-ences of pleasure."[501]

- One mother said her boy cried chronically for an entire year after circ.[502]

Circ Complications Overview

Medicine defines a complication as an unexpected problem that occurs soon after surgery. No law requires reporting complications, so there is no database of them, and estimates vary widely. H. Patel reported a 55% complication for circ,[503] but Jorgen Thorup et al. estimated it at only 2% to 10%.[504] One study estimates that the rate of severe circ complications requiring hospitalization was approximately 0.01%.[505]

Attorney Georganne Chapin notes that over 11% of pediatric malpractice lawsuits are for circ, usually for complications.[506] Pediatric surgeon David Gibbons, said that about 45% of complication cases require corrective surgery."[507]

Pediatric surgeon Daniel Shinhar lists five common types of circ complications, starting with the most frequent:

1. Bleeding
2. Infection
3. Penile damage
4. Narrowing of the urethra (which often appears later)
5. Asymmetrical remaining foreskin, which may be surgically corrected for cosmetic reasons[508]

These complications may be reported without mentioning circ as the proximate cause.[509] Likewise, when complications are treated in places other than those responsible for the original circ, the general inability to cross-link data in countries (such as the US) without unique personal identifiers often obscures the circ link.[510]

Late complications are almost never recorded as circ related. For instance, one study analyzed circ-induced pediatric surgery cases and found that 5% occurred 2 to 49 months after circ.[511] Another sign of the magnitude of the problem was that, of all outpatient visits (of all genders) to the pediatric urology department of one hospital during a 1-year period, 7% were for circ-related complaints.

As mentioned in the introduction, circ is deemed a minor surgery, and is thus often entrusted to medical students. In addition, a Canadian study found that most medical practitioners performing circ were poorly trained.[512] Sadly, Dr. Christopher Fletcher describes how some physicians are even expected to circumcise with no training at all—they learn by trial and error.[513]

Pediatric urologist Asseem Shukla reports that he does 50 to 55 circ "do-overs" every year (a second surgery to fix the first).

What follows is a list of the many potential complications of circ.

Infections Other Than UTIs or STIs

About two million infections are acquired annually in American hospitals, leading to 100,000 deaths.[514] The circ wound boosts the probability of getting these infections, which is especially dangerous because of multidrug-resistant bacteria, also called superbugs.[515] For example, a 2003 outbreak of the superbug methicillin-resistant *Staphylococcus aureus* (MRSA) in a hospital maternity ward resulted in three circumcised boys being infected.[516]

Van Howe and Robson implicated circ as a significant risk factor in a 2007 outbreak of MRSA in American cities.[517] And there was a case of necrotizing fasciitis (a flesh-eating bacterial disease) following circ.[518]

Sudden Infant Death Syndrome

Sudden infant death syndrome (SIDS) is diagnosed when an infant dies unexpectedly for unknown reasons.[519] It is the leading cause of death in US infants under 1 year of age, accounting for about 2,700 deaths per year.

Professor Eran Elhaik proposes that SIDS is the result of cumulative painful, stressful, or traumatic exposures that begin in utero and taxes neonatal regulatory systems. He suspects that circ is a factor because of the male predominance of SIDS (60:40)[520] and because states with higher circ rates have a higher male-to-female ratio of SIDS deaths. In general, the SIDS mortality rate is significantly correlated with circ.[521]

Bleeding

There are those babies who bleed so severely after circ that they may require transfusions,[522] but some still die from blood loss.[523] In one circ study, 2% of boys had to return to the hospital due to excessive bleeding.[524]

The reported incidence of postcircumcision hemorrhaging (bleeding) covers an extraordinary range across studies, from 0.08%[525] to 35%.[526] The differences may in part be explained by another study, which found that there is more bleeding from circ than is typically reported. The reason is that visual inspection of a baby's diaper is not an accurate representation of bleeding severity since super-absorbent materials manifest less blood on them.[527]

Urologist James Snyder comments, "It takes just a few diapers full of blood for an infant to die. Mohels are not equipped to handle this. Every few years there's a headline about a bleeding death from circumcision, but most cases aren't reported. And the death certificate will probably only report bleeding as the cause, not the circumcision which caused the bleeding."[528]

The Talmud mentions fatal bleeding following circ. Rabbi Judah decreed that the sibling of two brothers who died of bleeding after circ should not be circumcised.[529]

Vitamin K deficiency is sometimes observed in newborns, and some believe it is caused by blood loss due to circ.[530]

I interviewed a woman who said that her uncle bled to death from his circ. And her son got a severe infection from circ with the Plastibell device but fortunately survived.

Cancer

Circ increases the odds of certain types of cancer, though the rate is unknown. For example, 15 patients developed squamous cell cancer from their circ scars in just one region of Saudi Arabia.[531] And at the endnote is a case study of a penile tumor that developed after circ.[532]

Breastfeeding Disruption

Circ can possibly disrupt breastfeeding and impair maternal bonding.[533] One study demonstrated that most babies would not nurse right after they were circumcised, and those who did refused to look into their mothers' eyes.[534] Another study showed that circumcised boys breastfed less.[535] But yet another study maintained that circ did not affect breastfeeding. However, that study only looked at indirect measures of breastfeeding success, such as a lower incidence of jaundice.[536]

From all the above, circ likely does complicate breastfeeding.

Lopsided Foreskin

If the foreskin is removed asymmetrically, the appearance may be lopsided, and worse, might also create scarring and circ-induced phimosis. The disfigurement is sometimes called hypospadias or epispadias, which refers to the meatus not ending up at the tip of the penis. Circumcision clamps sometimes cause this. All of these problems likely require a second surgery.[537]

Fistulas

A fistula is a tunnel between body cavities that shouldn't be there, and circ sometimes causes it. With the powerful clamps that are used, it's not surprising that this happens. Fistulas can also occur from use of the Plastibell device or from postcircumcision stitches.[538] There are no statistics describing the rate of occurrence of circ-induced fistulas, but one study described 15 cases,[539] another delineated a procedure for repairing coronal fistulas,[540] and another gave a detailed description of one instance.[541]

Adhesions

Shaft skin remaining after circ may reattach to the glans during healing, especially if any of the mucous membrane of the inner foreskin is left. One study reported that 15% of circumcised boys have trouble with these, which are difficult to treat.[542] Corticosteroids have been tried but are ineffective.[543]

Another study reported on other dermatologic complications that can occur following circ, including a penile cyst, a penile skin bridge (when leftover foreskin adheres to the glans), and a buried penis (a penis that is covered by excess skin in the pubic area or scrotum).[544] One British man got extreme "buried penis" from circ and couldn't have sex.[545] At the endnote, is a link to an adhesion horror story that befell novelist Gary Shteyngart, written with his trademark sense of humor.[546]

Corona Obliteration

Sometimes circ causes considerable damage to the corona (rim at the base of the glans).[547] This has been known for centuries, as is written in the Mishnah (200 CE): "If [after circ] nothing is left of the corona, it's considered a severed penis, and he is prohibited from marrying a Jewish woman [presumably because someone with a severed penis can't procreate]."[548]

Necrosis

Necrosis of the penis means that most of its cells are no longer functional—it is "dead."[549] It has been known to happen, and the only "treatment" seems to be intentional amputation.

Amputation

One shocking type of circ accident is the partial or total amputation of the penis along with the foreskin.[550] The literature is filled with case reports.[551,552] Other than penile amputations as a cancer treatment or as elective transgender surgery, circ is probably the single largest cause of penile amputation in the US.[553] In one case, surgeons were able to reattach the penis.[554]

Improperly placed clamps are the usual cause of amputation. Sometimes, if just the glans is amputated, it can be reattached.

An infamous case is that of David Reimer, whose circ ravaged his penis so badly that it had to be amputated. He was raised as a female and later committed suicide.[555] And here's a recent case of circumcision-induced penile amputation in Israel (link at the endnote).[556]

Loss of Pheromones?

It has been hypothesized, but not proven, that the foreskin emits pheromones (gaseous sexual attractants).[557] Smell has been shown to play a role in human sexuality; for example, women are attracted to men whose immune system smell complements their own,[558] and men gave larger tips to lap dancers who were fertile, possibly being guided by smell.[559]

Paraboschi and Garriboli proposed that the frenulum produces a pheromone via apocrine glands.[560] Separately, Guest argued that the foreskin's sebaceous glands emit pheromones.[561] Fleiss and Hodges believe that foreskin pheromones are odorless but are still perceived by a woman's olfactory system.[562]

Opioid Addiction

Here is a title from a study in the journal *European Urology*: "An Opioid Prescription for Men Undergoing Minor Urologic Surgery Is Associated with an Increased Risk of New Persistent Opioid Use."[563] Circ was one of the surgeries mentioned.

Meatitis and Meatal Stenosis

Meatitis is an irritation of the meatus (peehole). Usually, meatitis which occurs immediately after circ can be treated with palliative treatments such as petroleum jelly and may go away on its own.[564] However, in the days following surgery, the exposed meatus can be irritated by urine, feces, or clothes. The ensuing inflammation narrows the hole and causes an obstruction called "meatal stenosis" (narrowing of the meatus).[565]

The possible symptoms of meatal stenosis are pain, urinary stream deflection, urinary frequency, and incontinence. Studies reported meatal stenosis rates of circumcised boys ranged from 7% to 20%.[566,567] The treatment is a surgery called meatoplasty, which enlarges the opening.

One of the biggest problems that has led to continuing high rates of US circ, is the Centers for Disease Control assertion that complication rates are negligible,[568] based on a study by El Bcheraoui et al.[569] But, as mentioned, other studies of just this one type of complication, meatal stenosis, reported rates of 7–20%.[570,571,572,573] This contradiction can be explained by understanding that meatal stenosis can take years to develop,[574,575,576,577] and El Bcheraoui et al. only analyzed complications after 180 days, yielding a tiny rate of .01%. In addition, the CDC ignored all the other complications that I listed above. Just as with the anesthesia issue, it only paid attention to one dubious study.

Circ can also cause meatal ulceration, an erosion of the meatus. Problems with the meatus can even lead to obstructive kidney disease.

At the endnote, is a link to a video of a case of a circumcised boy with severe meatal stenosis.[578]

Death

US Navy Rear Admiral Dr. Robert Baker estimated that at least 229 US babies die annually from hospital circ.[579] European Urology Focus reported that deaths from circ were often attributed to other causes.[580] Keeping that in mind, the rates reported in the following two studies are probably much higher: in South Africa, 400 circ deaths occurred over a six-year period,[581] and in Toronto,[582] the circ fatality rate was 0.0012%.

Why isn't this widely known? For one, inaccurate death certificates for children are common.[583] For example, if circ led to sepsis (blood poisoning) then the death certificate would have likely only mentioned sepsis, and not circ.[584,585] Other circ deaths might be disguised as surgical errors, infection, hemorrhage, cardiac arrest, stroke, reaction to anesthesia, or even parental neglect.[586] And coroners, who certify the cause of death, don't even need to be a medical doctor in some places in the US.[587] In other instances, death certificates have often listed misleading causes of death too. For example, the Love Canal poisoning with toxic chemicals in 1978 caused many cases of cancer, but the death certificates never mentioned the poisoning.[588] Finally, if parents want to sue for a circ gone wrong, they rarely have the resources to fight a hospital in court, and even if they do, the cases are often privately settled, with no disclosure of the outcome, so it will never be known that circ was the cause.[589]

But there's another long-term source of death from circ: suicide, a case of which I mentioned above. There are no statistics on this, but Georganne Chapman, CEO of Intact America, wrote about many suicides she knows of that are linked to despair over circ.[590]

Curvature of the Penis

The foreskin runs about halfway down the shaft, where its skin merges with the shaft. Thus, it can be difficult to determine where the foreskin ends and the shaft skin begins, especially when dealing with an infant's diminutive penis. Thus, circumcisers sometimes accidentally cut off shaft skin, too. This can lead to skin tightness which permanently curves the penis over time[591,592] and this happens to about 1% of circumcised men.[593] This curvature (called Peyronie's disease) can cause painful erections. Dr. James Snyder maintains that the cause is almost always circ.

Here's a testimonial from a 43-year-old man: "I didn't even know I'd been circumcised until I was 14. When I became erect, my penis would be pulled into a downward curve, which hurt every time. I thought this was normal. I developed erectile dysfunction."[594]

In 1995, the parents of a three-year-old boy won a $1.2 million settlement for removal of too much skin during their son's circ. Experts testified that the boy was likely to encounter problems in sexual functioning.[595]

Miscellaneous Possible Complications

- Keloids are fibrous scars that can arise from circ.[596]
- Sometimes, air sacs of circumcised babies' lungs can rupture from intense crying.[597]
- Cyanosis means that a body part turns blue because blood circulation has been cut off, and it has happened from circ.[598]
- Circ creates a loss of immune function in the penis since the foreskin contains thousands of lymphatic vessels and exocrine glands.[599]
- Acute ischemia (loss of blood supply) of the glans has happened. In one case, hyperbaric oxygen therapy successfully treated it.[600] Blood loss can also lead to gangrene, of which there are many reported circ-induced cases.[601]
- Circ has indirectly caused bladder perforation (because severe meatal stenosis blocked urine flow).[602]
- One study notes four cases of babies whose heart failed after circ.[603]
- The pain caused by circ may be so severe that babies vomit during the procedure.[604] At the endnote is a link to a video of a mother describing this.[605]
- Some circumcised men (like me) complain of having a cold penis. For testimonials, see the video link at this endnote.[606]

- Pus-filled cysts could form, and if they became infected might require additional surgery.[607]
- Pneumonia can occur after circ
- Liver or kidney failure can occur after circ
- Stitch tunnels (blackheads from sutures) can result after circ[608]
- At the endnote, is a link to a video about a mother testifying about her son, who got a hernia from his intense screaming following circ.[609]

———————

Finally, most of the medical issues I have reported in this chapter come from hospital circ, but in England, the medical board responsible for overseeing circ averaged four cases per year of significant problems from religious circ, including deformed penises and instances of emergency blood transfusions.[610]

Problems Later in Life

Sexual Complications during Heterosexual Intercourse

I'm going to discuss heterosexual sex in this section and gay sex in the next section.

Sexual problems may arise many years after infant circ, so proving cause and effect is not straightforward. Also, sexual pleasure is hard to measure; various scales for it have been attempted, but none is widely accepted.[611] Due to all these factors, almost all scientific papers ignore sexual loss resulting from circ.

Circ can remove the most erotic penile areas, each of which can trigger orgasm: the frenulum, ridge mucosa, and external foreskin fold.[612] In one survey, most intact men reported that the foreskin's to-and-fro movement over the glans was the ejaculation trigger.[613] The least sensitive foreskin parts are more sensitive than the most sensitive parts of the circumcised penis.[614] Thus some circumcised men struggle just to feel anything erotic during sex.[615]

The glans is composed of mucosal skin, similar to nipple skin, and as such, should be especially sensitive. But the circumcised man's perpetually exposed glans eventually loses almost all its sensitivity to touch, as reported in three different studies.[616,617,618] This is because by the time a circumcised male reaches his late teens, the skin on the glans will be up to 10 layers thick and its nerve endings smothered under layers of skin.[619] None of this layering occurs with intact men.

Therefore, it's inevitable that a circumcised man requires more vigorous and prolonged stimulation to trigger orgasm.[620] Overall, circumcised men experience significantly reduced sexual sensation,[621] since the intact penis is four times more sensitive than the circumcised penis.[622] These changes alter intercourse mechanics and have profound effects on women too, as I'll discuss in the next chapter.

Frisch et al. conducted the most comprehensive and elegant study of circ and sex. After controlling for confounding variables, they found that circumcised men were three times more likely to experience orgasm difficulties.[623] This replicated what Rowland found[624] when he did a robustness statistical analysis, which showed that circumcised men's difficulties were not explained by an excess of anxiety or depression in this group. This suggests that reduced penile sensitivity may, at least partly, explain circumcised men's sexual difficulties, an explanation that is supported by three neurophysiological studies.[625,626,627]

Circ increases the force required to penetrate by tenfold,[628] and 43% of circumcised men experience difficult penetration.[629] Three different studies showed that circ decreased sexual pleasure and reduced orgasm intensity.[630,631,632]

In an unhelpful study, Bossio et al. reported that penile sensitivity was not reduced by circ,[633] but the authors explained that they were only proving that the remaining penile parts after circ are as sensitive as they always were. This is like stating that if you amputate a toe, the rest of the foot would still be just as sensitive. The authors also admitted that "the circumcised penis glans was significantly less sensitive than the intact penis glans."[634]

Consider how sexual intercourse works for a male—maximizing pleasure hinges on a steadily ascending crescendo of erotic sensations culminating in orgasm. However, nerves don't easily conform to such a process. To grasp the problem, try this experiment suggested by O'Hara and O'Hara:

> "Run your finger lightly and slowly in a wide, circular motion around the underside of your wrist. You should notice pleasurable tingling sensations. Pause and lift your finger. Then begin anew, first slowly, but gradually speed up until you are going quite fast. Notice that the sensations are strong at first, but eventually recede until the area goes numb. This is because nerves need time to recharge before they refire."[635]

The erotic evolution solution: Use two sets of nerves during intercourse. Some fire on thrusting in, others fire on pulling out. On the instroke, the touch-sensitive nerves of the exposed glans and foreskin are stimulated. On the outstroke, the foreskin covers the coronal ridge and corona, so the touch-sensitive nerves have time to rest, as the vagina bears down and stimulates the penile area containing pressure-sensitive nerves. Thus, a male has continuous pleasure sensations as he ascends to orgasm.

Strip away the foreskin and this dynamic is lost. A fully circumcised man may have to have a staccato rhythm of stop and start during intercourse to allow his only remaining nerves (the pressure-sensitive ones) to reset.

There are also pressure-sensitive nerves at the penile base and pubic mound, which in an intact male are more frequently stimulated because of much shorter strokes. (We'll see why later.)

Given all of these problems, it's predictable that erectile dysfunction (ED) is a common consequence of circ, at a rate 4.5 times that of the intact male.[636,637,638,639,640] In one of these studies, before adult circ 19% had ED, but after circ 30% had greater, mild, or moderate ED, and 35% had weakened erectile confidence.[641] Dr. Christopher Fletcher comments about ED, "I prescribe many more times Viagra for circumcised guys than for normal men."[642]

Two studies associated circ with increased premature ejaculation,[643,644] which is when a man comes too fast and experiences significantly less pleasure from the orgasm. Sex physiologist Roy Levin calls anything less than 2.5 minutes thrusting time "probable premature ejaculation."[645]

As long as a thousand years ago, Rabbi Isaac Ben Yedaiah wrote, "A woman will passionately desire an uncircumcised man because he thrusts inside her a long time due to his foreskin which is a barrier against ejaculation. Thus, she achieves orgasm first. But a circumcised man will perform quickly, coming as soon as he inserts his glans."[646]

However, two other studies have found that circ reduced incidence of premature ejaculation.[647] I think at least part of the confusion occurs because, as explained above, circumcised men rely on different nerves than intact men, and the different nerves types may require different thrusting times and rhythms, so it's not useful to equate the two situations.[648]

Four separate studies found that the best orgasms could only be achieved with a foreskin. Two reached this conclusion by measuring the lack of triggering in circumcised men of the penilo-cavernosus reflex (which is responsible for deep erogenous sensation and ejaculation).[649,650] No study found that circ improves sensitivity or erectile function.

———————

Another way we can determine the effects of circ on sexuality is by observing circumcised men who restored their foreskins by stretching it over extended periods, as in ancient Greek times. The slow stretch is often called tugging, which is a more accurate term than "restoring" because nothing will bring back the erogenous nerves that were cut away. Improvement in glans sensitivity is the goal of this practice,[651] and the glans also becomes softer.[652] At the endnote is a link to one website that offers guidance.[653] And at the next endnote, is a link to a podcast relating one Jewish man's experience with tugging.[654]

Another option is using surgery to revive glans sensitivity. One study describes how this reconstruction was done by essentially cutting and stitching together the remaining foreskin until it covered the glans.[655] Another study focused on surgically lengthening the frenulum with excellent results.[656] Possible risks of these types of surgeries are inflammation of the glans, infection, and excessive bleeding.[657]

One company is even experimenting with regrowing foreskin by engineering the patient's own cells to regrow foreskin.[658]

———————

Still another way to ascertain circ's sexual damage is by studying men who underwent circ as adults, possibly as a treatment for phimosis, or for conversion to Judaism. Here are the results:

- One study found that on average there was a loss of pleasure from masturbation or intercourse.[659]
- South Korea presents a unique opportunity to study the effects of circ since millions of males have been circumcised there after becoming sexually active, because, as mentioned, it was a habit picked up from Americans. A majority of these men reported diminished sexual pleasure, and some had erectile pain from skin adhesions.[660]
- Denniston reported similar results of males circumcised in adulthood.[661]
- In an *Ha'aretz* survey, 70% of men circumcised as adults reported less enjoyment of sex following circ.[662]

Circumcised men required more effort to achieve orgasm, and a higher percentage experienced unusual sensations (burning, prickling, itching, or tingling and numbness of the glans) and described discomfort, pain, and numbness of the shaft.[663]

I should note that in any study there will always be men who report better sex after circ. However, as noted above, many of the sexual problems occur over time, such as numbing of the glans, and keratinization, and these would likely not have been observed at study time.

Over a lifetime, a circumcised penis is also more prone to abrasion, bleeding, and pain, either from trauma such as bumping into things, or from intercourse.[664] I had these problems on a number of occasions.

A couple of women I interviewed noted that it's harder to give a circumcised man a hand job, and none said it was easier.

One published survey found that 55% of circumcised men said they were dissatisfied with their sex lives and 39% admitted to disinterest in sex. Some said they had relatively good sex but complained that "it's not all it's cracked up to be" and wondered "if I'm missing something."[665]

Circumcised men's reduced ability to achieve a satisfactory orgasm results in a loss of marital satisfaction.[666,667,668,669,670] Also, men's mortality risk declines as the frequency of orgasm increases, with a whopping 50% reduction for those at the highest frequency levels.[671] Finally, semen has been shown to have an antidepressant effect for females, so frequent (unprotected) sex has an important health benefit for them too.[672]

The healing power of sex is amazing, though all too temporary. During sex, a person who has a stutter may lose it, amputee phantom limb pain may disappear, and even the muscle spasticity of cerebral palsy may calm down.[673] An active, pleasurable sex life is correlated with better cognitive functioning in all genders. The people who experienced the most pleasure had larger hippocampi, which are tied to memory and other brain functions. High sexual pleasure also correlates with lower blood pressure, less cardiovascular disease, and better emotional health: less anxiety, higher self-esteem, better sleep, and less depression.[674]

Having an orgasm at least three times a week halves a man's likelihood of heart disease, and having more ejaculations is correlated with less of a risk of prostate cancer,[675] which is men's most common cancer. The leading explanation for this is the "prostate stagnation hypothesis," which says that the buildup of fluid in the prostate is an irritant that increases cancer risk.[676,677]

In the Netherlands, sex is seen as a human right. As such, disabled citizens can get government funding for legal prostitutes up to 12 times a year. Reports show this has significantly reduced depression and suicide rates among people with disabilities.[678]

Of course, loss of the entire foreskin will be more damaging than circ that retains the frenulum.

Here are some statements from boys circumcised as teenagers:

- "Circumcision is like going from color vision to seeing in black and white."[679]
- "I was much less sensitive and required more stimulation to reach erection."[680]
- "Erections during recovery were very painful. Sex became very problematic. Plenty of insecurity, loneliness, and addiction to porn. [I got into] tantra, the spiritual side of sex, to heal."[681]

And let's hear from some men circumcised as adults:

- "Awful loss of sensitivity and function afterward.[682]
- "Intercourse now is like washing your hands with gloves on."[683]
- "I enjoy no glans sensations; orgasm requires painful thrusting."[684]
- "Before circumcision, orgasms were reached easily (but not prematurely), and were intense enough to make my knees give way if I was standing. My glans dried out and became much less sensitive, as did my frenulum. I now masturbate with lubrication and achieve orgasms with extreme difficulty. They are still pleasurable but are much less intense. I married at age 23, and throughout the next 17 years, I often had trouble climaxing in intercourse due to lack of glans sensation. I never could climax through fellatio, which had not been a problem before."[685]
- "Since I had my penis circumcised I lost 80% of my penis's sensitivity and have no response to my wife's vaginal movements. I take so long

to orgasm that I irritate my wife's vagina, even though we use lots of lubricant. She complains that my penis often feels hard and painful without the soft foreskin. She only reaches orgasm now with her own hand stimulating her clitoris. I have little sensitivity and thus no buildup of feeling or response during intercourse, so I just pound harder and faster in desperate hope of reaching orgasm."[686]

_____

A misleading recent meta-analysis on the effects of circ on sex, which is supposed to look at all the literature in the area, only considered one study by a well-known pro-circ author[687] and ignored all the data I presented above. So, of course, it concluded that circ does not affect sexual sensitivity or satisfaction.[688]

To summarize: Heterosexual circumcised men can still enjoy sex, but less so than intact men. That's if they can have sex at all, and don't have erectile dysfunction, curved penis, or other significant circ issues. It's also assuming their partners aren't in such pain that they're unwilling to participate.

If circ causes so many sexual problems, why was it even approved? It comes back again to medicine's disregard of pleasure issues in favor of focusing on pathology. There is an analogous situation with the birth control pill, which can permanently damage a woman's libido and yet is still on the market. As neuroendocrinology professor Kim Wallen notes about the pill, "The US Food and Drug Administration doesn't consider behavior, and in particular sexual behavior, to be something they're concerned about."[689]

Circ and Gay Men

Gay men have a strong preference for sex with men with intact penises.[690] Childhood circ does not appear to affect gay men's sexual behavior. However, when they were circumcised at later ages they tended to engage in, and prefer, receptive anal intercourse, with the implication that being the active partner was now less pleasurable.[691]

Masturbation Difficulties

Masturbation is a natural behavior, common among male nonhuman primates.[692] Psychologist Jesse Bering believes that humans are the most masturbatory of all species, due to our advanced ability to imagine events, such as erotic scenes.[693]

In a study of adult men, 63% had more difficulty masturbating after circ.[694] Circumcised men are more likely to use artificial lubrication for masturbation[695] while an intact man can simply manipulate his foreskin without additional aid. In fact, some intact males (and no circumcised males) can stimulate themselves to orgasm without even touching their penis.[696] Given these facts, it is likely that circumcised men masturbate less, though no study has demonstrated this.

But masturbation has many health benefits: it increases serotonin and dopamine, improves sleep, reduces stress, improves the fitness of sperm, tones the pelvic floor muscles, improves sexual intercourse performance, and reduces pain.[697] Masturbation also increases penile blood flow, which over times helps prevent erectile dysfunction.[698] And a man's orgasm frequency correlates with more immunoglobulin A (an immune system component). So, any procedure that reduces masturbatory frequency is detrimental to a man's health.

Shortening of the Penis

Circ shortens the length of both the flaccid and erect penis, by an average of 1 cm.[699] It also reduces the girth. Most men find this quite an undesirable outcome.

Slow Healing

Heat hastens the resolution of minor glans abrasions incurred from sex or perhaps unwelcome contact with an obstacle like a drawer. With a foreskin, the penis stays warmer, promoting healing of these irritations. Also, circumcised men have a much greater probability of a penile burn.[700]

Discomfort Wearing Clothes

Some circumcised men experience discomfort from underclothes.[701,702]

Aesthetic Harm

Does the circumcised penis look better or worse? There is no definitive data. In my discussions with women, there was an even split in preference. Many interviewees had never had sex with an intact man. As one Jewish woman put it, "I guess it depends on what you get used to."

Autism?

In a study by Frisch and Simonsen, Danish boys circumcised in their first 10 years had a shocking 54% increased risk of autism spectrum disorder. Even more disturbing was that the risk increased up to 83% for boys circumcised in the first four years of life.[703] These remarkably high figures are only correlational, and more studies need to be done before reaching any conclusions.

DOCTORS' STATEMENTS

Statements from circumcising doctors reveal troubling experiences:

- "We typically circumcised in a locked soundproofed room. As I cut one baby, there was a blood vessel where there shouldn't be one. The baby bled and bled. We called in five other doctors to help and finally had to transfuse the baby. We never told the mom what happened. That is what you did to cover up these things. It still goes on."

- "I was consulted regarding one baby who was just circumcised. He had lost all his penile skin all the way down to the abdomen. It was horrible and will be an automatic lawsuit. This boy will be scarred for life."[704]

- Urologist Adrienne Carmack noted, "Believing circ is not harmful is not an 'opinion.' The hundreds of boys I have seen who needed surgery to repair problems caused by their circumcision are real. The men who lost more parts of their penis than the foreskin are real. The thousands of adult men saying they wish they hadn't been cut are real. Not recognizing that circumcision is harmful is either ignorance or denial."[705]

- Dr. Christopher Fletcher conducted an anonymous survey of physicians who circumcise. More than half said they circumcised for the money and didn't believe it had any benefit.[706]

- A survey showed that only about one-third of the physicians thought that the benefits of circ outweighed the risks.[707]

- One doctor bluntly admitted after doing a circumcision, "There's no medical reason to do this."[708]

A recent study that was brave enough to challenge circ orthodoxy in America said, "Nontherapeutic circumcision has little or no high-quality medical evidence to support its overall benefit. Moreover, it is associated with rare but avoidable harm and even occasional deaths. There is no medical justification for performing circumcision prior to an age that [a boy] can assess the known risks and potential benefits and give or withhold informed consent."[709]

To demonstrate the effect of circ on populations, we can look to Australia, where was a large decline in circ rates—from 40% in the early 1980s to 10% in 2006. Correlated with that drop, there was a 50% reduction in child deaths over the same period.[710] Of course, this only suggests circ might be related to more deaths, as many other factors could be involved.

MEDICAL SUMMARY AND CONCLUSION

In summary, the medical benefits of circ are questionable, and the risks are significant, especially considering the lifelong loss of pleasure. On my website, linked at this endnote,[711] is a concise list of the pros and cons of medical circ.

CHAPTER FOUR

Intact Men and the Women Who Love Them

Female Perspectives on Male Circumcision

The Frisch et al. sex study mentioned above found that for the average woman, sexual intercourse with an intact man was significantly more fulfilling, with fewer orgasm difficulties. Strikingly, female pain during intercourse was four times greater with circumcised men.[712] As one woman testified, "[During sex with a circumcised man] my vagina tightens up so much that intercourse is painful or virtually impossible."[713] The rest of this chapter will explain why this happens.

While direct internal anatomical observations of coitus are limited to a solitary (but famous) MRI study published in the *BMJ* (formerly known as the *British Medical Journal*),[714] much can be deduced from behavioral reports, surveys, and logical inferences.

Removing the foreskin changes profoundly alters the dynamics of sexual intimacy impacting the thrust's gliding action, smoothness, force, depth, duration, rhythm, and lubrication—factors that shape both partner's pleasure. Below is the breakdown.

THE FORESKIN'S SILKEN GLIDE

O'Hara and O'Hara analogized the mechanics of heterosexual intercourse with this experiment. "With an intact man, the foreskin is the main point of contact

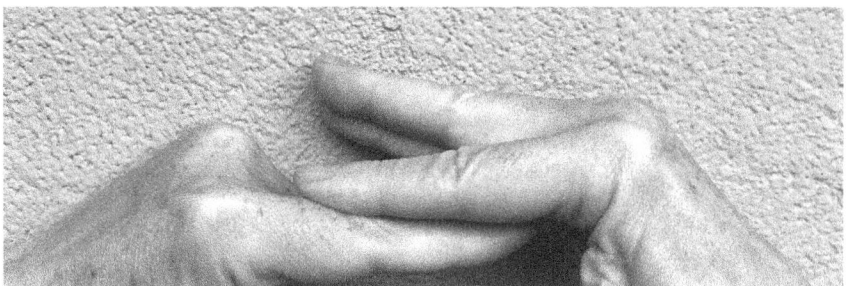

FIGURE 10. *Finger analogy of sexual intercourse*

with the vaginal opening, and the penis slides under it. To understand how this works, take the index finger of your left hand and point to your right.

"Take the fingertip of your right index finger and place it, flat, on top of your left finger's center knuckle. Your left finger is the penis; its loose knuckle skin is the foreskin, your right finger is the vaginal wall, its fingertip is the vaginal opening.

"Move your left finger back and forth to the extent your knuckle skin allows. Notice that although the 'penis' is moving in and out, it is gliding on its own skin, so there is no friction with the vagina.'"[715]

Thus, no foreskin, no glide.

FRICTION'S FLAME

In a survey, many women expressed laments such as, "A circumcised penis creates more friction. The intact penile foreskin stays in the same place, while the penis inside it moves back and forth."[716] The vagina also has interior ridges which can comfortably mesh with the foreskin.

THRUST FORCE

A circumcised male has a fairly numb glans, so he thrusts as hard as he can to generate sensation. It doesn't seem too rough to him, because many of his sensory nerves have been cut, but it may cause irritation to his partner.

When he thrusts, he primarily stimulates pressure-responsive nerves, called Pacinian corpuscles, which are in the deeper penile tissues. They are less sensitive, and so they require more force. In addition, the missing frenulum would have resisted forceful action, because if it's jerked on vigorously, it overstretches, creating male discomfort.[717]

As one woman put it: "Circumcised men work awfully hard to orgasm and need a lot more violent thrusting. I thought sex was painful until I did it with a natural man."[718]

THRUST DEPTH

An O'Hara and O'Hara survey noted that 73% of women reported that circumcised men thrust harder and deeper, using more elongated strokes, and are less in contact with the mons pubis and clitoris (because the penis pulls back farther so that it can thrust harder).[719] This reduces female stimulation.

Some survey responses were as follows:

- "Circumcised men don't feel close because they are too busy moving in and out instead of staying in and moving around."[720]
- "When I'm on top, I use short, rubbing, jiggling movements. My circumcised partner doesn't find this satisfying and keeps trying to do longer strokes."[721]
- "The circumcised man always pulls his body away from my clitoris. I keep trying to pull him closer, but he pulls away. It's annoying, like being in a wrestling match. My natural (intact) partner always stays close to my genitals, giving me the consistent pressure I need to attain orgasm."[722]

INTERCOURSE LENGTH OF TIME

In the O'Hara and O'Hara survey, 42% of survey respondents stated that their circumcised partners had to work too hard at achieving orgasm. Some women might consider lengthy intercourse a positive, but probably less so if the man seems to be struggling.

A man who takes too long to climax experiences the opposite of premature ejaculation; medically it is called delayed ejaculation, which is defined as taking more than 30 minutes to climax (from the start of intercourse) or becoming too tired to go on. Frequent delayed ejaculations can cause significant stress and impact personal relationships.[723] With sex, timing is everything.

THRUST LUBRICATION

In a circumcised man, the corona (rim of the glans) pulls the vaginal secretions from the vagina when the shaft pulls back. This doesn't happen with an intact penis because the foreskin serves as a plug. In addition, the foreskin's smegma provides lubrication too.

THRUST RHYTHM

One key point is that the thrusts of an intact man produce more frequent rhythmic contact with the clitoris because, as I explained, the circumcised man may stop and start.

The O'Hara and O'Hara survey also yielded an astounding 70% of women who said that with circumcised men, they often wished to just get sex over with. With intact men, 91% want it to continue. These figures are so high that they definitely need to be replicated to be trusted.

Here are some more survey comments:

1. "My husband had his foreskin restored. We both now appreciate his control and staying power. And I no longer experience soreness, even with prolonged intercourse."[724]
2. "The circumcised man goes too fast or slow. With my intact partner, intercourse was rhythmic, like dancing gracefully together. We were so in tune with each other. I felt like I was melting into him."[725]
3. "It's generally harder to bring circumcised men to climax, which can take the joy and closeness from the encounter, leaving me feeling frustrated and unsatisfied."[726]
4. An RN writes, "The circumcised penis is less capable of responding to sexual stimulation and transmits less pleasure than an intact one. It is easier to bring an intact man to full erection and maintain it, and I receive a much more enjoyable rainbow of vaginal sensations and a more exciting object to fellate."[727]
5. "You get double-motion action with an intact man; it's the best."[728]

Miriam Pollack notes that circumcised men often lose their sensitivity just as perimenopause may decrease a woman's vaginal lubrication. Sexual difficulties at that point may be totally ascribed to the woman when it's actually likely a mix.[729]

O'Hara and O'Hara reported that women had a greater chance of having a vaginal orgasm with intact men.[730] A different study showed that women who have sex with a circumcised man have 19% less vaginal lubrication.[731] I wonder how many women have been described as "frigid" when their sole problem was their circumcised partner?

Another issue is that some women's sexual response may partly depend on her perception of her partner's pleasure, which is, as we've learned, diminished by circ.[732]

Here is one poignant story: "My boyfriend and I were very happy and compatible in bed. But I refused to get married until he was circumcised—and he gave in. That operation destroyed our life together. Before, he had fabulous staying power, but after circ he would have an orgasm in five minutes and leave me high and dry. Sex became painful. Twice, I had infections from chafing. We no longer speak."[733]

Blogger John Erickson writes, "A prostitute who's had intercourse with thousands of men told me that intercourse with a circumcised vs. intact man were two entirely different experiences; she could always sense circumcised status, and circ men took longer to ejaculate, and they had to work at it."[734] A porn actress I interviewed expressed similar sentiments.

CIRC AND MOTHERHOOD

Circ may also consternate some mothers because it violates their instinct to protect their child, as several women authors have commented.[735,736]

I would also ask, how much trust has the infant lost in his mother? We know babies can distinguish their mothers from other women within hours of birth and discern emotions within days.[737] And as mentioned, circ may cause problems with nursing and even eye contact.[738]

Finally, I'll conclude this chapter with this question: Why do we have ribbed condoms? They mimic foreskin ridges.

CHAPTER FIVE

Penis Facials Anyone?

Foreskin Finances

How much does circ cost? Ritual circ is generally a private transaction with little available data, so here I will discuss hospital medical circ. Statistics cited are for the US, unless mentioned otherwise.

JALOPIES FOR PATIENTS

Hospital circ costs vary widely depending on where it was done, what insurance was involved, and whether there were complications. Also, cost estimates sometimes just refer to the procedure, whereas other data cite the entire patient bill, which includes the cost of the hospital room and other ancillary expenses.

The doctor's fees alone usually run from $500 to $2,500. There are also possible expenses for hospitalization, laboratory fees, medications, supplies, and other incidentals.[739] The total hospital bill, even without complications, can easily exceed $3,000.[740] But complications can increase the tab. About 3% of boys require surgical revision,[741] with an average price of $1,727, just for the extra surgery.[742] One case even cost $17,000.[743]

The average cost of pediatric circ in a doctor's office (outside of a hospital) is $2,003 in 2024.[744]

Another hidden patient cost of circ is for long-run items such as erectile dysfunction drugs, sexual lubricants for the dried-up penis, and even psychotherapy costs.

MERCEDES FOR DOCTORS

Dr. Timothy R. B. Johnson, a professor of obstetrics and gynecology, describes circ as a money machine for the pediatricians at his hospital who can do as many as five per hour. The charge was about $175 per circ in 2017[745] (just for the procedure, not the hospital room or other costs.)[746] The current circ record holder is Dr. Pinhas Gonen, who did 63 circumcisions in one day.[747]

In 2021, one physician reported earning $600 per circ.[748] Another physician crowed, "I love doing circumcision—they make my Mercedes payments."[749] Pediatricians also see circ as a way of establishing a lasting relationship with parents.[750]

When the British National Health Service stopped paying for circ in 1949, the rate dropped to less than 1%. And in the US, Medicaid payments correlate with the rate of circ.[751] In the 17 states where Medicaid does not cover circ,[752] it is 24% less common.[753] And as soon as insurance coverage for circ was dropped in California, rates plummeted 28%.[754]

Several medical clinics advertise both performing circ and treating erectile dysfunction, thus fixing the very condition they contributed to—the perfect business model.

LAMBORGHINIS FOR THE HOSPITAL

The foreskin removed during a brit is typically buried. However, the circ industry's shocking big secret of medical circumcision is that the hospital often sells cells, usually fibroblasts, from the removed foreskin. Fibroblasts are one of the most important repair cells of the body. Biotechnology companies use them to create products that are used for wound healing, tissue engineering, and anti-aging products. So, medical circ is just organ harvesting by another name.

Patients and their guardians are not aware that this happens and receive none of the profit. More on the ethics of this later.

It's not clear how much hospitals are paid for foreskins. However, companies do buy them from hospitals and then process and sell them, usually as vials containing about 500,000 foreskin cells. The vials run from $199 to $500.[755] Examples of these vial sellers are Invitrogen—whose vials cost $339 each,[756] and American Type Culture Collection—at $440 each.[757]

Below are the detailed uses of foreskins and their fibroblasts.

Research

Fibroblasts have been used to grow robotic fingers,[758] obtain induced pluripotent stem cells, diagnose *Clostridium difficile*, test drug toxicity, study disease development of various pathogens, and study cellular physiology.[759] And in a bizarre experiment, entire human foreskins were grafted onto mice in the quest to develop the Gardasil 9 HPV vaccine mentioned above.[760]

Skin Grafts

Fibroblasts secrete collagen proteins that maintain the structural framework for various tissues. They also play a key role in wound healing. The products are often called "neonatal human dermal fibroblasts," which is a euphemism for foreskin-derived fibroblasts. To give you an idea of the interest in them, a 2020 Google search yielded an astonishing 698,000 results, mostly for companies selling foreskin-derived products.

For example, foreskin-derived Apligraf is touted as a living cell skin substitute. It has a myriad of skin graft uses; for example, reconstructing a woman's vagina after cancer, which costs $2,000 for each six-inch circle.[761] Similarly, Dermagraft is used to treat diabetic foot ulcers.[762] It seem likely that patients don't even know that these are foreskin-derived products.

So hospitals can possibly profit from every end of the circ process: the procedure itself, repairing complications, foreskin sales, and then treating medical conditions with foreskin products.[763]

Cosmetics

The most profitable use of foreskins is for cosmetics, which can sell for as much as $1,000 a vial. For example, Allergan's SkinMedica produces foreskin-derived skin-cream products[764] popularized by talk shows. Allergan has a staff of 250 employees generating $80 million in annual sales.

One treatment is called a "penis facial" or "Hollywood EGF facial" (because the process involves the application of a foreskin-derived epidermal growth factor, or EGF serum). A study funded by the manufacturer found that daily applications of EGF serum improve skin texture, pore size, red spotting, and wrinkles."[765]

Driven by celebrity mentions, the $650 penis facial had a *two-year* wait list in 2019.[766] You can also get a "hydrafacial," which incorporates foreskin fibroblasts for $249 per treatment. It is offered at many spas.[767]

Profit from Invisible Foreskins

Another way that hospitals make money on circ is to charge for it even if it wasn't done. Pat Palmer, founder of Medical Billing Advocates of America, says that hospital billing errors are par for the course, and sometimes bills for male circumcision are sent to parents of newborn girls, or to boys who didn't get circumcised. Gynecologist Dr. Ghosh notes that these "mistakes" for procedures not rendered are common, because patients often don't examine their bill's complicated details.[768] And some hospitals just issue a bill with no itemization at all. For example, in his superb exposé book, *The Price We Pay: What Broke American Health Care—and How to Fix It*, Dr. Marty Makary describes how it took him many months of battling a hospital's bureaucracy (and a $25 fee) just to get an itemization for a friend's bill.[769]

In the first-of-its-kind reporting, intactivist Anthony Losquadro revealed how hospital foreskin sales work. The size of the business is jaw-dropping. Organogenesis Holdings Inc., a public company valued at $367 million (in May 2024) buys foreskins from hospitals and produces the two graft products mentioned above. Three well-known hospitals that have contracts with Organogenesis are Tufts Medical Center, Boston University Medical Center, and the Iowa Clinic. The contracts have a confidentiality clause which demands that parents not to be told about the foreskin sale. Hospitals maintain the foreskin is medical waste and therefore becomes a possession of the hospital. Further, Losquadro writes, "Organogenesis pays doctors and hospitals . . . for their . . . cozy business relationship. In one year, Organogenesis paid $1.3 million. One doctor received $80K annually, which included payments for giving speeches, and compensations for travel, lodging, and food. In other words— free vacations."[770]

With all these profit streams, you can see why circ is an incredible $5.7 billion industry in the US (in 2020).[771]

Given that circ is a hospital's pot of gold, it's no wonder that mothers are often coerced into circumcising their sons. A survey by Intact America showed that mothers were asked an average of eight times if they wanted circ for their son, and 78% of mothers had their sons circumcised if health providers asked, compared to only 45% of mothers who were not asked.[772]

Some mothers' statements are as follows:

- "I was badgered repeatedly with lines such as, 'He won't feel it. It's quick; it's better for him.'" See a link to her video at the endnote.[773]
- "I was shamed for refusing circ."[774]
- "When my son was born, I was asked at least four times in a single day if we had decided on circ. Nobody offered any explanation. My answer was repeatedly no, only to hear a mumbled reply about cleanliness, parental preference, and UTI prevention. The last time they barged in and exclaimed, 'Okay, it looks like he's ready for circumcision!' I banged back 'NO THANK YOU!' and the nurse turned and walked out. If I hadn't been on guard, they would have tricked me into it."[775]
- When intactivist Marilyn Milos's son was born the doctor described circ like this, "It doesn't hurt, only takes a minute, and will protect your son throughout his life."[776] That's an economical three lies in one sentence.

Hospitals manipulate parents in other ways: Hospital circ forms for mothers in labor are often presented at a moment when they are least likely to read them. One mother said: "I was asked three times while in the hospital if we wanted him circumcised, and I proudly said 'No!' every time." Another mother similarly reported.[777] As a father, Anthony Losquadro was also strongly pressured but resisted.[778]

Moreover, in the US, some cultures do not practice circ and some parents do not speak English, so these groups might not even understand what the word circumcision means. There also are many reports of boys being circumcised in hospitals against their parents' wishes.[779] That often only comes to light when there are significant surgical complications that lead to court cases, such as the three examples at the following endnotes, which led to plaintiffs receiving up to

$1 million.[780,781,782] Also, even when consent is obtained, it only has to be from one parent, and is often not "informed" consent, meaning the parent is not apprised of the risks.[783] More on this point later.

Another sneaky tactic is pro-circ websites designed to look like purely informative science. But if you read the fine print, usually in small font at the bottom of the page, you see that the website is just a vehicle for advertising a doctor group that does circ. I found three of these type online.

The Morality of Foreskin Sales

Using circ for medical research violates The Declaration of Helsinki, a set of ethical principles widely regarded as the cornerstone document on human research ethics,[784] and multiple other human rights treaties.[785] This leads to the next chapter.

CHAPTER SIX

Rights or Rites?

The Ethics and Legality of Circ

Circ pits parents' rights to act for their child against infant boys' rights to physical integrity.

Many people believe that removing healthy tissue from an infant should only be permissible if there is an immediate medical indication. The American Academy of Pediatrics Committee on Bioethics states that interventions that can safely wait until the child can provide his own consent should be delayed until that consent can be obtained.[786] Apparently, one committee doesn't talk to another at the AAP, because in the AAP's 2012 policy statement on circ, which I covered above, this issue wasn't mentioned. The AAP's circ policy statement also ignored yet another of its own reports, also cited above, that recommended reducing the pain from procedures as much as possible.

Ninety medical, legal, ethics, and human rights scholars issued a paper concluding that circ is morally wrong since there is no reason for doing a medical procedure when there is no immediate threat, combined with the fact that here are less harmful ways of avoiding future problems.[787] Similarly, bioethicist Brian Earp maintains that children have a right to body autonomy and should decide about body alterations when they are of the age of consent.[788]

Another issue is that circ practitioners often ignore the protocols for informed consent. And those doctors who explain the procedure to their patients greatly understate its risks. As Harvard ethicist Harriet A. Washington notes, consent needs to address what the average patient would "need to know to be an informed participant in the decision."[789] With circ, consent covers neither the short-term or long-term side effects, nor the financial incentives for the physician and hospital.

Attorney J. Steven Svoboda notes, "The basic human rights principle that the human body should not be used to make money without the patient's permission is well established. Circumcision violates four core human rights documents—the Universal Declaration of Human Rights, the Convention on the Rights of the Child, the International Covenant on Civil and Political Rights, and the Convention against Torture."[790,791]

CIRC IN COURT

A California appeals court held that an unnecessary surgery constitutes harm, even if it is performed perfectly.[792] So it can be argued that since circ is unnecessary, it is deemed harmful under the law.

In 2020, a lawsuit was filed in Massachusetts demanding that Massachusetts Medicaid stop paying for infant circ because federal and state regulations require that all services paid for by Medicaid be medically necessary, and circ is just elective cosmetic surgery.[793,794] A Massachusetts state trial court responded to the lawsuit and ruled that MassHealth, the state health agency, violated state law[795] by paying for medically unnecessary infant circumcisions.

A 2021 lawsuit against the AAP alleged that fraud led to a botched circ in New Jersey in 1997. The lawsuit contended that the AAP had several undisclosed biases, including a financial one, and made false policy claims in its 1989 policy report.[796]

A 2024 bill to ban Medicaid coverage of circ failed in the New Hampshire state house.[797]

———

One group of legal and medical professionals wrote, "Circumcision is a complex, 150-year-old multibillion dollar-per-year fraud."[798] Nevertheless, no US doctor has ever faced liability for doing a normal circumcision.

A 1996 federal law banning female circumcision illustrates the intricacies of American law. In 2008, a judge declared the law unconstitutional on the grounds that female circumcision is clearly a crime, and only states can pass criminal laws (unless they affect interstate commerce).[799]

In the United Kingdom, female circumcision is banned under the Female Genital Mutilation Act of 2003, but there is no law covering male circ.

In Malawi (formerly part of Rhodesia) 312 minors have sued a circumcising organization for assault, battery, pain, suffering, and disfigurement.[800]

MEDICAL ASSOCIATIONS' VIEWS

As I mentioned before, not one medical association in the world recommends circ. In Israel, circ is viewed as a religious ceremony, so the Israel Medical Association does not pass judgment on it. A similar situation exists in Muslim-majority countries.

Here are the medical associations that outright condemn circ for minors:

The Danish Medical Association (87% of Danes favor banning circ)[801]

The Royal Dutch Medical Association[802]

The Royal Australasian College of Physicians, the Royal Australasian College of Surgeons, the Urological Society of Australia and New Zealand, and Australian state health departments[803]

The Nordic Ombudsmen for Children

The German Pediatric Association[804]

The British Medical Association[805]

Canadian Paediatric Society[806]

Places that have discussed banning circ include Finland, Iceland, Denmark, Sweden, and San Francisco, though none ultimately passed new legislation.[807,808,809] I am against a legal ban, because it might traumatize the Jewish and Muslim communities, with many Jews seeing it as the kind of existential threat they have faced since the time of the ancient Greeks. Moreover, prohibition would likely just drive the practice underground, and would be almost impossible to enforce, since religious circ is usually a private ceremony.

A more constructive approach focuses on more education, mandatory expansive informed consent, and stopping government insurance coverage of the practice.

Legal scholar Prof. Michael Freeman even argues that Jewish and Muslim circ constitutes a human right. For some boys, circ is more than a medical procedure; it could be seen as a crucial part of cultural and religious identity. Even delaying the procedure to adulthood could be very stressful.[810] Following this line of thinking, would a Jew or Muslim feel out of place with his peer group if it became known that he wasn't circumcised? Possibly so, though I know of no instances where this has happened. I interviewed a rare intact Jew and also an intact Muslim. Both never had a problem with their foreskin status.

There are two other issues.

First, should the parents be informed about the foreskin sale? As a guide, the Code of Medical Ethics of the American Medical Association requires that a physician should declare his economic interests.[811] The hospital secret sale of foreskins violates the principle of autonomy, which requires that patients have the right to make informed decisions about their own bodies and medical treatments. Moreover, it violates the principle of beneficence, which requires that medical interventions should be done for the benefit of the patient, not for the profit of others. Finally, there is a clear conflict of interest for medical professionals, who may have a financial incentive to promote circ and to downplay its risks and complications.

A second question: Shouldn't the circumcised person have rights to the profits on the sale of his foreskin?

The book *Mine!: How the Hidden Rules of Ownership Control Our Lives* does not discuss circ but mentions similar cases where patients' cells were used for profit without their knowledge, such as the famous case of Henrietta Lacks's cancer cells, described in the book *The Immortal Life of Henrietta Lacks*. Researchers have used clones of her cells in countless experiments since they were collected in 1951. Lacks's daughter complained about not receiving compensation,[812] and finally, in 2023, 72 years after the cells were taken, she received an undisclosed sum.[813]

In the US, ownership of bodily resources is mostly not regulated except in certain specific instances, such as a ban on selling kidneys. The various levels of government—federal, state, county, and local—all have different, and sometimes contradictory, regulations.[814]

A fair and practical legal remedy would be to pay royalties to the patient for use of his foreskin cells, as has been suggested in similar cases of body parts usage.[815]

Another issue is that medical protocols are often violated when it comes to circ. For example, it is standard to require consultation between the primary care physician (in this case, usually a pediatrician) and the surgeon before any surgical intervention. Yet obstetricians routinely circumcise the newborn without consulting the pediatrician.[816] Finally, soliciting patients for cosmetic surgery is considered unethical, but it's regularly done for circ.

CHAPTER SEVEN

The Unkindest Cut

American Medicine's Stubborn Stance on Circ

With so much evidence against circ, why aren't more US physicians abandoning it? Here are some possible reasons.

FEAR OF DEFYING ESTABLISHED GUIDELINES

Medical knowledge doubles every 3.5 years,[817] so most working physicians understandably rely on the policies of authoritative bodies. American circ guidelines are built on the edifice of the 2012 American Academy of Pediatrics Circumcision Policy Statement, discussed above, which reported that circ benefits outweigh the risks.[818] Two years later, the CDC affirmed the report as its policy too.[819]

In a podcast interview, lead author of the AAP Policy Statement, Andrew Freedman, described how he circumcised his son. The host, Wendy Zukerman, was shocked, because until that point the evidence discussed in the program seemed poor. Freedman said he did it because of Jewish tradition.[820] Shouldn't the AAP statement have disclosed this bias?

In a separate interview, Dr. Freedman disclosed another questionable issue. He said that when the report stated that the benefits of circ outweigh the risk, it wasn't exclusively referring to medical benefits but also included other benefits, such as religious ones. If this is the case, the report should have stated that explicitly.

Other problems with the report:

- It ignores all the important foreskin functions
- The quantity and quality of short-term circ complications are mostly unknown, so a risk/reward analysis is meaningless.[821]
- The significant long-term consequences of circ, especially loss of sexual pleasure, discussed above, are not even considered.[822]
- It gives credence to the African studies on HIV, which are critiqued above.
- It brushes aside the issue of pain, even to the point of ignoring its own AAP perspectives on it, which are issued in a different report.
- It ignores psychological and emotional harm.

In a paper published in the journal *Pediatrics*, 38 European physicians denounced the AAP circ policy statement, writing that the benefits are "questionable, weak . . . and do not represent compelling reasons for surgery before boys are old enough to decide for themselves."[823]

I note that the policy expired in 2017. Follow the link at the endnote to view the report, which clearly states, "This policy automatically expired."[824] Since expiration, the policy has not been reinstated, nor are there any plans to do so.

Many US hospital committees only consider whether a procedure is "clinically acceptable" before recommending it, and circ falls in that category. It doesn't matter if there are better ways of doing medicine; the committees can always justify their decision by that label.[825] And a doctor who bucks the system risks being labeled a "disruptive physician," which could lead to loss of hospital privileges.[826]

One surprising new form of censorship might come from artificial intelligence (AI) programs. As of this writing in 2024, Claude 3 Opus, created by the company Anthropic, is the AI program with the highest accuracy rating, according to some sources. I queried Claude 3 about my circ stances. It admonished me that I shouldn't speculate about circ and called some of my assertions "alarming." Instead, it suggested that I should just rely on "trusted sources" such as the American Academy of Pediatrics. And popular AI program ChatGPT warned me that my query may violate its guidelines (probably because it involved sexuality).

CLINICAL DETACHMENT

With regular exposure to illness and/or death, it is understandable that doctors strive to maintain a certain level of detachment. But you can take a good thing too far.[827] For example, one woman I spoke with told me that she insisted on observing her son's circ, over the objections of the two doctors who were in charge of the procedure. She was appalled to see that their attention during the cutting was mainly focused on discussing their golf game.

IGNORANCE OF FORESKIN ISSUES

Here are some examples of more invisible foreskins, even in recent times:

2004—Of 90 American medical textbooks and anatomical models less than one-third featured an intact penis.[828]

2010—American medical texts portray circumcised penises as normal and may define the foreskin as "the part removed by circumcision."[829]

2021—*Men's Health: An Introduction* has a section on male urogenital anatomy that minutely explores every male part except the foreskin.[830]

2021—*The Every Body Book* has only two illustrations of penises, both of which are missing foreskins.[831]

2024—My urologist has an extremely detailed diagram of male genital anatomy on his wall—with no foreskin.

Resistance to foreskin education is part of American culture's shunning of knowledge about sex itself, where we still retain vestiges of Victorian sensibilities. Even as late as the 1960s, medical sexual discussions were somewhat taboo. For example, a popular medical physiology book had no entry for penis, erection, or ejaculation, and physiology courses didn't cover orgasm or even arousal. In 1966, when Masters and Johnson published their seminal *Human Sexual Response*, they got a lot of hate mail, and medical journals rejected their work. In the 1970s, the FBI even put a researcher named Vern Bullough on its list of dangerous Americans, for promoting legalization of oral sex and publishing articles about prostitution.[832]

In 1964, Kalcev incorrectly wrote that all boys should retract their foreskins, even if they had to force it.[833] It seems that some ideas, like this one, become so entrenched that it is difficult to overturn them later. Here are the results of that thinking over the years, based on various studies:

1981—A study found that physicians often gave no guidance or gave incorrect advice regarding the foreskin. The study also included parental reports of physicians wrongly and forcibly retracting their son's foreskin during infancy.[834]

1982—A study showed that both physicians and mothers believed the 1964 false Kalcev conclusion.[835]

2007—Astonishingly, 31 out of 32 medical texts (erroneously) wrote that the foreskin should retract by age 5 or earlier.[836]

2011—Only 2% of doctors and med students fully understood intact infant hygiene, which mainly focuses on retraction and cleaning. Many male doctors themselves are circumcised, and therefore might consider the foreskin abnormal.[837]

2020—One study showed that 49% of medical residents had not been taught intact penile care, and only 60% gave advice to parents, and what they said varied greatly.[838]

2023—Over 75% of foreskin problem diagnoses were incorrect, mainly due to retraction ignorance.[839] Similar poor education has been shown for nurses.[840]

In 2022, the American Academy of Pediatrics finally set up an official policy on foreskin retraction, saying "Forcing the foreskin to retract before it is ready can cause severe pain, bleeding, and tears in the skin."[841] Maybe this will start to help.

In September 2023, Intact America conducted a nationwide survey regarding infant male circumcision. The reaction of the respondents was this:

- 39% said that they don't know what happens during circ.
- 46% were not aware of circ complications.[842]

So the American public is ignorant of foreskin issues too, which further doesn't incentivize doctors to make changes either.

CHANGE IN MEDICINE IS DIFFICULT

Nothing better illustrates medicine's resistance to change than the case of Ignaz Semmelweis, MD. In 1840, many women died from childbirth from what was called childbed fever. Semmelweis was a keen observer, and noticed that when midwives delivered babies, as opposed to doctors, there was almost no illness. He concluded that the fever was coming from something doctors did. In those days, doctors had to examine cadavers regularly to maintain their skills. Semmelweis realized that the sickness came from "poisoning" from the cadavers and proposed that doctors should wash their hands before delivering babies.

This might seem innocuous, but it incensed members of the establishment, who hounded Semmelweis until he was driven into a mental health facility where he was put in a straitjacket, kept in a dark room, and beaten mercilessly. He died two weeks later.[843]

Similar resistance to change exists in the medical profession today; for example, as mentioned above, outmoded pain techniques are used for tracheostomies. Dr. Suchi Saria, founder of Medical AI company Bayesian Medicine put it, "Every time I walk into a hospital, I feel like I've stepped 10 or 20 years into the past."[844]

PUBLICATION BIAS

As discussed before, Dr. Morten Frisch had a tough time getting anti-circ papers published. Van Howe notes that American medical journals will readily publish pro-circ articles but will often reject anti-circ ones.[845] And in general, medical journals tend to only publish studies with positive outcomes.[846]

Another problem with publication is that once a false study gets published, it is repeatedly cited even after there's overwhelming evidence to the contrary. And the rebuttals are often published as "letters to the editor," which usually don't carry the same weight as the original study and are far less noticed.[847]

FEAR OF BEING LABELED AN ANTISEMITE

Frisch said about a review of his circ study: "I [previously] never had vicious and indecent comments, accusing me of racism and dishonesty. I had many papers published with no trouble, but when I added the variable of circumcision, the trouble started."[848]

FINANCIAL INCENTIVES

The US government relies on medical organizations to set medical policy, which leads to biased decisions, since circ is quite profitable.

Another type of bias is pro-circ research conducted by individuals who had incentives to promote circ, such as a pro-circ meta-analysis[849] whose authors had undisclosed publication motives. For instance, one author was part of a pro-circ lobbying organization whose members were circ doctors, and another author had a patent pending for a circ device.[850]

HARD-TO-BREAK INERTIA

Although some physicians remain skeptical of circumcision, their ongoing practice of it still suggests to patients that it holds value. Briggs gives the example of a hospital that stopped performing inpatient circ, and, although several physicians still offered outpatient circ services, the rate dropped considerably even for the outpatients.[851] In other words, patients pay attention to doctor's behavior as cues to the best medical practices.

CHAPTER EIGHT

Tools of the Trade

Circ Instruments

THE SHIELD

The Jewish shield, described above, causes some bleeding, which is seen as a halachic advantage because, for circ to be valid, there must be blood (possibly as evidence of periah, or perhaps just as a badge of sacrifice). Even in the rare case of someone born without a foreskin, halacha demands that a mohel extract a token amount of blood to simulate circ. However, while Yahweh is said to require blood, doctors hope to avoid it. So other instruments were invented.

THE GOMCO CLAMP

The Goldstein Manufacturing Company invented the Gomco clamp, mentioned above, in 1935, to make circ easy, efficient, and, especially, bloodless. It is the most widely used hospital circ tool, chosen by 67% of doctors.[852]

Rabbi Eliezer Waldenberg, an Orthodox rabbi known for both his compassion and his erudition, wrote, "The moment the clamp is placed on the body of the child, his entire body turns blue from the intense pains that are caused."[853] Bravo, Rabbi Waldenberg, for being a rare rabbi to sound the alarm! A clamp is likely significantly more painful than a quick slice, although no study has proven this.

One advantage of freestyle circumcision using just a scalpel and shield is that the mohel can accurately deal with any anatomical irregularities. Clamps use a one-size-fits-all approach, which can cause problems.

THE MOGEN CLAMP

In 1955, Rabbi Harry Bronstein invented a different type of clamp called the Mogen clamp.[854] It was easier to use than the Gomco, but most importantly, it allowed a trickle of blood to flow, thus satisfying halachic requirements. Ten percent of American physicians used the Mogen as of 2010.[855]

Circ using the Mogen was reported to be less painful than that using the Gomco[856]; however, it had a higher risk of harming the glans. Between 2000 and 2011, the US Food and Drug Administration received 139 reports of problems caused by circ clamps, especially the Mogen, including 51 injuries.[857] Litigation against Mogen led to bankruptcy, but some practitioners still use it.

There is debate about the use of clamps among Orthodox Jews.[858]

THE PLASTIBELL

The Plastibell is a piece of plastic inserted under the foreskin that causes it to become necrotic (dead) and fall off after 7–10 days. According to one study, it is "a safe technique with minimum complications,"[859] but another study reported an 8% complication rate.[860] However, remember that these are only the immediate complications. I noted above how the Plastibell was one of the noted causes of fistulas and secondary phimosis, both of which can occur years later.

Another study found that the Plastibell saved time and had similar results to "freehand" circ.[861] The Plastibell is the second-most popular circ instrument in hospitals, used by 19% of doctors.[862]

THE CIRCULAR STAPLER

The circular stapler is a newer Chinese device that has a saw to cut the foreskin, and stapler to close the wound. It appears to have reasonable results but has not been widely adopted.[863]

PREPEX

The PrePex is similar to the Plastibell. It is FDA-approved but not available in the US. It was designed as a simple-to-use device, primarily for African circ.[864]

LASER

Huang et al. recently proposed using a laser for circ, describing it as a "novel, less complicated, easy, and less painful alternative procedure."[865] So far, it has not been adopted.

HEATING CAUTERY

A study conducted in Iraq reported that heating cautery (burning off the fore-skin using heat conduction from a metal probe) was the most common circ technique used there, but it is unknown in the West. The study reported that it caused a shockingly high 40% rate of meatal stenosis and cautioned against using it.[866]

Here is a table of circ method comparisons from the United Nations:[867]

Method	Advantages	Disadvantages	Comments
Dorsal slit	Can be performed in any hospital or clinic equipped with standard surgical instruments	Requires more surgical skill than other methods	Can be undertaken by skilled surgeons who do not regularly perform circumcision
Plastibell	Simple technique Can be performed using EMLA cream anaesthesia	Requires a stock of different sizes of device Plastibell stays attached for 3–4 days until it drops off May require second clinic attendance to have the bell removed	Suitable for clinics dealing with large numbers of babies
Mogen clamp	Technique using one-piece instrument, which is simple to use; simple to teach Produces a crushed welded edge, which does not need suturing	Risk of partial amputation of glans if device is not applied carefully Risk of glans being buried by cross-adhesions	Although suturing is not usually needed, it may be on occasion, thus surgical skills must be available in clinics where these devices are used
Gomco clamp	Simple technique; can be performed with EMLA anaesthesia Produces a circular crushed welded edge that does not need suturing	Clinic needs to have a set of Gomco clamps with different bell sizes Multipart device, with risk that parts will be lost or damaged Parts not readily interchangeable between different clamp sets	Although suturing is not usually needed, it may be on occasion, thus surgical skills must be available in clinics where these devices are used
Metal shield	Simple technique using one-piece instrument (the shield that protects the glands), which is simple to use; simple to teach even to laypeople Can be performed anywhere and with any amount of (neonatal) foreskin	Risk of partial amputation of glans, if circumciser is not careful	Used by mohels and could be found in several formats: one-time use or multi-use with sterilization

FIGURE 11. *Advantages and disadvantages of common methods of circ. Used with permission of the United Nations.*

In a survey of mohels, no Reform Jewish mohels used the shield, but they were willing to use the Gomco clamp because they don't believe in the necessity of blood. Jewish circ methods have evolved throughout history. No mohel who performs the procedure today does it like was done in biblical times.[868]

CHAPTER NINE

Conclusion

I make a firm recommendation against circ based on all the evidence, but what you do is, of course, up to you.

I will leave you with a statement of principles that I like, from a group called Doctors Opposing Circumcision:[869]

> We envision a world free from forced genital cutting, one where children's rights are respected and their wholeness protected.

Statement of Principles

- **Anatomy and function**—The foreskin is a normal, healthy, valuable part of the human body, with multiple functions, both protective and sexual. Every effort should be made to protect and preserve this unique tissue.

- **Medical non-necessity**—There is no medical reason for infant circumcision. Infant circumcision is "non-therapeutic" because there is no disease or injury requiring treatment. No medical organization recommends circumcision as a routine procedure for all males. The foreskin is no more prone to problems than any other part of the body. If needed, conservative treatments are available and effective. Disease is best prevented by attention to simple hygiene and proven behavioral risk factors.

- **Risks and harms**—Circumcision entails a wide array of physical risks and emotional impacts, and detrimentally alters sexuality. These harms vastly outweigh any claimed benefit.

- **Medical ethics and human rights**—Circumcision is an irreversible, medically unnecessary procedure that removes a normal, healthy body part from a non-consenting patient. As such, it violates every fundamental principle of medical ethics—beneficence, non-maleficence, autonomy, justice, and proportionality. It also violates numerous human rights principals, especially those pertaining to protecting children.

- **Role of the health professional**—D.O.C. urges all health care professionals to take their ethical obligations to patients seriously, by refusing to participate in infant circumcision and taking an active professional role to end it. Doctors should be healers, not brokers of harmful cultural practices.

- **Genital autonomy**—All children—male, female, and intersex—should be protected from medically unnecessary, non-consenting genital alteration. This includes gender assignment surgeries on intersex children, and "genital normalizing" surgery in the case of hypospadias and epispadias. D.O.C. endorses the 2012 Helsinki Declaration of the Right to Genital Autonomy.

- **Adult choice**—Adults too should not be subjected to medically unnecessary, non-consenting alterations of their genitals. Adults choosing elective genital alteration must be free from coercion, and fully informed of the attendant risks, harms, and losses.

- **Gender equality**—As in many other countries, females have been protected from genital cutting by U.S. federal law since 1997. Boys and intersex children deserve the same protection for their genital integrity and autonomy.

- **Breastfeeding**—Breastfeeding is very important to child health. The pain and trauma of circumcision interferes with the initiation of breastfeeding, as well as with the mother-child relationship.

- **Religion and culture**—All children, regardless of culture or religion, have the right to be protected from bodily harm. A child's right to bodily integrity outweighs parental preference, cultural norms, or religious rituals. (*Prince v. Massachusetts*, U.S. Supreme Court)

Acknowledgments

Thanks go to the following:

- My publishing coach, Mike Daniels, who was exactly the person I needed to help me hold everything together. He is a masterful publishing navigator.
- My other book coach, Karma Bennett, whose wizardry proved that I had a marketable product.
- My beta readers, who unselfishly gave freely of their time to critique my manuscript: Dr. James Schneider, Dr. Jeffrey Levy, Dr. Farhad Ahmed, J. Steven Svoboda, Hector Nolle, Kristen Caven, Lisa Braver Moss, and Michael Watts.
- C. Daniel Miller, the Copyright Detective, whose adept guidance in navigating the labyrinth of permissions was indispensable in protecting my work and peace of mind.
- My talented illustrators: Chynna DeSimone (interior) and Julie Cohn for her watercolor cover. You can see more of Julie's fine art at https://juliecohnfineart.com.
- The organization Bruchim for welcoming Jews who question circ.
- Shut Up & Write volunteers who hosted the many writing sessions I attended for eight years.

Selected Bibliography of
Online Resources

WEBSITES

My own website: https://kennethlipman.com/
Bruchim: https://www.bruchim.online/
Intact America: https://intactamerica.org/
Genital Autonomy America: https://www.gaamerica.org/
Doctors Opposing Circumcision: www.DoctorsOpposingCircumcision.org
Circumcision Information and Resource Pages: www.cirp.org
Mothers Against Circumcision: www.mothersagainstcirc.org
Attorneys for the Rights of the Child: www.arclaw.org/
Circumcision Resource Center: www.circumcision.org
National Organization of Restoring Men (NORM): www.norm.org
Foregen: Regenerating the foreskin http://www.foregen.org
National Organization to Halt the Abuse & Routine Mutilation of Males
    (NOHARMM): www.noharmm.org
Circumstitions: www.circumstitions.com
Foreskin photos and more: www.foreskin.org
Genital Autonomy Legal Defense & Education Fund: www.Galdef.org

RESOURCES FOR JEWS OPPOSED TO INFANT CIRCUMCISION:
Bruchim: https://www.bruchim.online/

SELECTED BIBLIOGRAPHY OF ONLINE RESOURCES

www.beyondthebris.com
www.cutthefilm.com
www.celebratingbritshalom.com
https://www.circinfo.org/Jews_against_circumcision.html
Footage of a bris with commentary from the subject: https://www.youtube.com
/watch?v=VJ8Kt6Vu4oE

VIDEOS OF JEWISH MEN UNHAPPY
ABOUT BEING CIRCUMCISED:

https://www.youtube.com/watch?v=GVO6YzROkZE
https://www.youtube.com/watch?v=FCuy163srRc

Endnotes

1   Another practice from that era that defied common sense was doctors' endorsement of cigarettes, even to pregnant women. One ad stated, "More doctors smoke Camels than any other cigarette." Little, B. (2018). "When Cigarette Companies Used Doctors to Push Smoking," History Magazine, https://www.history.com/news/cigarette-ads -doctors-smoking-endorsement.

2   Perera, Caryn L., et al. Safety and efficacy of nontherapeutic male circumcision: a systematic review. *Ann Fam Med.* Jan-Feb 2010; 8(1):64–72, https://doi.org/10.1370 /afm.1073.

3   UNAIDS, Joint United Nations Programme on HIV/AIDS. 2012. Neonatal and child male circumcision: a global review (World Health Organization) (2012).

4   Al-Mayoof, Ali F., Esmaeel Almushhadany, Osama, Joda, Ali E., Kamil Mohammed, Mohammed. Evaluation of risk factors for secondary phimosis in children. *International Journal of Surgery Open* 2020/01/01; 24:69–72, https://doi.org/10.1016 /j.ijso.2020.04.003.

5   Frisch, Morten, Earp, Brian D. Circumcision of male infants and children as a public health measure in developed countries: A critical assessment of recent evidence. *Glob Public Health.* 2018/05/04; 13(5):626–641, https://doi.org/10.1080/17441692.2016.11 84292.

6   John, Timothy. Nurses of St Vincent: Saying NO to Circumcision (1994), https:// www.youtube.com/watch?v=Csaal-MqXB4.

7   Real, Terrence. *I Don't Want to Talk About It: Overcoming the Secret Legacy of Male Depression—Kindle edition by Real, Terrence.* Scribner; 1999. p. 22, https://amazon .com/Dont-Want-Talk-About.

-Overcoming-ebook/dp/B000FC0Q0C/ref=sr_1_1?crid=LNUHDYAJJ7G4&
dchild=1&keywords=i+don%27t+want+to+talk+about+it+terrence+real&qid=
1624733216&sprefix=i+don%27t+want+%2Caps%2C222&sr=8-1.

8   JT. Not Just a Flap of Skin. *skinforeblogspotcom* blog. 2009. www.skinfore.blogspot.com.

9   Panati, Charles. *Sexy Origins and Intimate Things: The Rites and Rituals of Straights,
     Gays, Bi's, Drags, Trans, Virgins, and Others*. Kindle Edition. 2012. loc. 1365, https://
     www.amazon.com/dp/B00AN959CW#detailBullets_feature_div.

10   Erickson, John A. 33 Photographs of The Intact Adult Male Foreskin. 1994, http://
     www.sexuallymutilatedchild.org/33.htm.

11   Gollaher, David. *Circumcision: A History of the World's most Controversial Surgery*.
     Basic Books, A Member of the Perseus Books Group; 2000. p. 5.

12   Berry, Carl D., Jr., Cross, Roland R. Urethral Meatal Caliber in Circumcised and
     Uncircumcised Males. *AMA Journal of Diseases of Children*. 1956; 92(2):152–156,
     https://doi.org/10.1001/archpedi.1956.02060030146007.

13   Cold, Cc; J. Taylor. The Prepuce. *Br J Urol*. 1999; 83(1):34–44.

14   http://gethelpwithjsj.blogspot.com/2009/09/great-first-aid.html.

15   Montagu, Ashley. *The human connection*. 1979, p. 47, https://books.google.com
     /books/about/The_human_connection.html?id=IZFRAQAAIAAJ.

16   Fleiss, Paul, Hodges, Frederick. *What Your Doctor May Not Tell You About
     Circumcision*. Hachette Book Group; 2002. p. 2.

17   https://15square.org.uk/.

18   Fleiss, Paul, Hodges, Frederick. *What Your Doctor May Not Tell You About
     Circumcision*. Hachette Book Group; 2002. p. 2.

19   Ball, Peter. A Survey of Subjective Foreskin Sensation in 600 Intact Men. In:
     Denniston G. C. HFM, Milos M. F., ed. *Bodily integrity and the Politics of
     Circumcision*. 2012.

20   Earp, Brian David, https://x.com/briandavidearp/status/1721095242693144975.

21   Personal Communication with James Snyder, MD. 2021.

22   Ball, Peter. A Survey of Subjective Foreskin Sensation in 600 Intact Men. In:
     Denniston G. C. HFM, Milos M. F., ed. *Bodily integrity and the Politics of
     Circumcision*. 2012.

23   Guest, Christopher. A Historical and Medical Critique of Circumcision. Accessed
     March 25, 2016, https://www.youtube.com/watch?v=XwZiQyFaAs0&list=PLKuasL
     inBzLvg-s777BUtAX23LTdDfU6g&index=39&t=0s.

24   Paraboschi I., Garriboli M. Functions of the Prepuce. *Normal and Abnormal Prepuce*.
     Springer, Cham; 2020:67.

25   O'Mara, Shane. *In Praise of Walking: A New Scientific Exploration*. W. W. Norton and
     Co.; 2020.

26   Ritter, Thomas J. *Say No to Circumcision!: 40 Compelling Reasons Why You Should
     Respect His Birthright and Keep Your Son Whole*. 2020. p. 11–12.

27   Lakshmanan, S. Parkash S. Human prepuce: some aspects of structure and function.
     Indian Journal of Surgery. 1980; 44:134–137.

28   O'Hara, K., O'Hara, J. The effect of male circumcision on the sexual enjoyment of the
     female partner. *BJU Int*. Jan 1999; 83 Suppl 1:79–84, https://doi.org/10.1046/j.1464
     -410x.1999.0830s1079.x.

29 Fink, Kenneth S., Carson, Culley C., DeVellis, Robert F. Adult circumcision outcomes study: effect on erectile function, penile sensitivity, sexual activity and satisfaction. *J Urol*. 2002; 167(5):2113–2116.

30 Tygenhof, Eric. Urologist explains the FACTS about newborn and infant circumcision, https://www.youtube.com/watch?v=iZ64pqWZRW8.

31 Goldman, Ronald. *Circumcision, The Hidden Trauma : How an American Cultural Practice Affects Infants and Ultimately Us All: Ronald Goldman: 9780964489530: Amazon.com: Books*. Vanguard; 1997. p. 39.

32 Sex and Circumcision—An American Love Story—by Eric Clopper. 2019, https://vimeo.com/316275787.

33 Ahmed, A., Jones, A. W. Apocrine cystadenoma. A report of two cases occurring on the prepuce. *Br J Dermatol*. Dec 1969; 81(12):899–901, https://doi.org/10.1111/j.1365-2133.1969.tb15971.x.

34 Weiss, G. N., Sanders, M., Westbrook, K. C. The distribution and density of Langerhans cells in the human prepuce: site of a diminished immune response? *Isr J Med Sci*. Jan 1993; 29(1):42–3.

35 Flower, P. J., Ladds, P. W., Thomas, A. D., Watson, D. L. An immunopathologic study of the bovine prepuce. *Vet Pathol*. Mar 1983; 20(2):189–202, https://doi.org/10.1177/030098588302000206.

36 Sex and Circumcision—An American Love Story—by Eric Clopper. Clopper, Eric. 2019, https://vimeo.com/316275787.

37 Circumcision, Task Force on. Circumcision Policy Statement. *Pediatrics*. 1999; 103(3):686–693, https://doi.org/10.1542/peds.103.3.686.

38 yourwholebaby.org. Images, https://www.yourwholebaby.org/the-intact-penis-page

39 Ritter, Thomas J. *Say No to Circumcision!: 40 Compelling Reasons Why You Should Respect His Birthright and Keep Your Son Whole*. 2020. p. 11–12.

40 Morris, Brian J., Wamai, Richard G., Henebeng, Esther B., et al. Estimation of country-specific and global prevalence of male circumcision. *Popul Health Metr*. 2016; 14:4, https://doi.org/10.1186/s12963-016-0073-5.

41 World Health Organization. *Male Circumcision—global trends and determinants of prevalence, safety and acceptability*. 2007.

42 Goldman, Ronald. *Circumcision, The Hidden Trauma : How an American Cultural Practice Affects Infants and Ultimately Us All*. Vanguard; 1997. p. 110.

43 Jacobson, Deborah L., Balmert, Lauren C., Holl, Jane L., Rosoklija, Ilina, Davis, Matthew M., Johnson, Emilie K. Nationwide Circumcision Trends: 2003–2016. *Journal of Urology*, https://doi.org/10.1097/JU.0000000000001316.

44 Cohen-Almagor, Raphael. Should liberal government regulate male circumcision performed in the name of Jewish tradition? *SN Social Sciences*. 2020/11/09; 1(1):8, https://doi.org/10.1007/s43545-020-00011-7.

45 Zambrano Navia, Mateo, Jacobson, Deborah L., Balmert, Lauren C., et al. State-Level Public Insurance Coverage and Neonatal Circumcision Rates. *Pediatrics*. 2020/11/; 146(5), https://doi.org/10.1542/peds.2020-1475.

46 wisevoter.com. Circumcision Rate by State, https://wisevoter.com/state-rankings/circumcision-rate-by-state/.

47   Theoharakis, Matthew, NewYork-Presbyterian Morgan Stanley Children's Hospital, New York N. Y., Feldman, Evin, et al. Circumcision. *Pediatrics In Review*. 2024; 43(12):728–730, https://doi.org/10.1542/pir.2022-005536.

48   Zambrano Navia, Mateo, Jacobson, Deborah L., Balmert, Lauren C., et al. State-Level Public Insurance Coverage and Neonatal Circumcision Rates. *Pediatrics*. 2020/11; 146(5) https://doi.org/10.1542/peds.2020-1475.

49   Wikipedia. Circumcision in Africa. 2022, https://en.wikipedia.org/wiki/Circumcision_in_Africa.

50   Lawal, T. A., Olapade-Olaopa, E. O. Circumcision and its effects in Africa. *Transl Androl Urol*. Apr 2017; 6(2):149–157, https://doi.org/10.21037/tau.2016.12.02.

51   Fleiss, Paul, Hodges, Frederick. *What Your Doctor May Not Tell You About Circumcision*. Hachette Book Group; 2002. p. 2.

52   Oh, S. J., Kim, T., Lim, D. J., Choi, H. Knowledge of and attitude towards circumcision of adult Korean males by age. *Acta Paediatr*. Nov 2004; 93(11):1530–1534, https://doi.org/10.1080/08035250410030018.

53   Wikipedia. Tuli (rite), https://en.wikipedia.org/wiki/Tuli_(rite).

54   WikimediaCommons. Global Map of Male Circumcision Prevalence at Country, https://commons.m.wikimedia.org/wiki/File:Global_Map_of_Male_Circumcision_Prevalence_at_Country.svg.

55   Morris, Brian J., Wamai, Richard G., Henebeng, Esther B., et al. Estimation of country-specific and global prevalence of male circumcision. *Popul Health Metr*. 2016; 14:4, https://doi.org/10.1186/s12963-016-0073-5.

56   Matar, Lea, Zhu, Julia, Chen, Robert T., Gust, Deborah A. Medical risks and benefits of newborn male circumcision in the United States: physician perspectives. *J Int Assoc Provid AIDS Care*. Jan-Feb 2015; 14(1):33–39, https://doi.org/10.1177/2325957414535975.

57   YouGov Survey, https://today.yougov.com/(popup:search/circumcision).

58   https://www.babycenter.com/4_will-you-circumcise-your-son_1546.

59   Undark Magazine. Snip or Skip? The Complicated Debate Over Circumcision. @undarkmag. Updated 2024-01-01, https://undark.org/2024/01/01/contested-science-circumcision/

60   Gollaher, David. *Circumcision: A History of the World's most Controversial Surgery*. Basic Books, A Member of the Perseus Books Group; 2000. p. 5.

61   Lev, Gid'on. Five Foot Six and Circumcised: CT Scan Uncovers Mummy of Pharaoh. *Haaretz*, https://www.haaretz.com/archaeology/five-foot-six-and-circumcised-ct-scan-uncovers-mummy-of-pharaoh-1.10498672.

62   Friedman, David M. *A Mind of Its Own: A Cultural History of the Penis*. Free Press; 2001. p. 92, https://www.amazon.com/dp/B003719FSM/ref=dp-kindle-redirect?_encoding=UTF8&btkr=1.

63   Fairfield, Jason, https://x.com/JasonFairfieldo/status/1705017259452731902.

64   Gollaher, David. *Circumcision: A History of the World's Most Controversial Surgery*. Basic Books, A Member of the Perseus Books Group; 2000. p. 5.

65   Herodotus. *The Histories*. The Penguin Classics. p. 116.

66   Gollaher, David. *Circumcision: A History of the World's Most Controversial Surgery*. Basic Books, A Member of the Perseus Books Group; 2000. p. 5.

67   Ahmed, Lieutenant Colonel Said. *Practical Surgery*. Young Medicos Organisation Publication; 1958. p. 156.

68   Edwardes, Allen. Erotica Judaica: A Sexual History of the Jews. Julian Press; 1967. p. 26.

69   Kirsch, Adam. *The People and the Books*. Norton; 2016. Loc. 384, https://books .google.com/books/about/The_People_and_the_Books.html?id=hMBojwEACAAJ.

70   Aronson, Louise. *Elderhood: Redefining Aging, Transforming Medicine, Reimagining Life*. Bloomsbury Publishing. loc. 1594.

71   Wikipedia. Olympic Games, https://en.wikipedia.org/wiki/Olympic_Games

72   Milius, Susan. First, Protect Today's Forest. *Science News*. (July 3 and July 17, 2021):27.

73   Chabad. Search for the word sacrifice in the Torah, https://www.chabad.org/search /results.aspx?scope=63255&searchword=sacrifice.

74   Berman, Samuel A. *Midrash Tanhuma-Yelammedenu*. KTAV Publishing House; 1996, https://books.google.com/books/about/Midrash_Tanhuma_Yelammedenu.html?id =WLOi9vWEzTEC.

75   i24 News. Was Pharoah circumcised? YouTube; 2022.

76   Kirsch, Adam. *The People and the Books*. Norton; 2016. Loc. 384, https://books .google.com/books/about/The_People_and_the_Books.html?id=hMBojwEA CAAJ.

77   4 Ever Green. 10 Uncontacted Lost Tribes That Never Evolved. YouTube, https:// www.youtube.com/watch?v=AvDE83uasS8.

78   Goldfarb, Kara. Five-Year-Old Albino Child Beheaded In Ritual Killing. *@atinteresting*. Updated 2018-05-16, https://allthatsinteresting.com/albino-child-murder-mali.

79   Glick, Leonard B. *Marked in your flesh : circumcision from ancient Judea to modern America*. Oxford: Oxford University Press; 2007. p. 32–33.

80   Personal communication with Dr. David Paslin.

81   Romberg, Henry MD. *Bris Milah: A Book About the Jewish Ritual of Circumcision*. Feldheim Publishers; 1982. p. 191.

82   Ahmed, Lieutenant Colonel Said. *Practical Surgery*. Young Medicos Organisation Publication; 1958. p. 156.

83   Kirsch, Adam. *The People and the Books*. W. W. Norton & Company; 2016. Loc. 384, https://books.google.com/books/about/The_People_and_the_Books.html?id= hMBojwEACAAJ.

84   Stavrakopoulou, Francesca. Why was Circumcision IMPORTANT in Ancient Israel? YouTube, https://www.youtube.com/watch?v=J7UagGacaJs&t=21s. YouTube.

85   Edwardes, Allen. Erotica Judaica: A Sexual History of the Jews. Julian Press; 1967. p. 30.

86   Edwardes, Allen. Erotica Judaica: A Sexual History of the Jews. Julian Press; 1967. p. 38.

87   Edwardes, Allen. Erotica Judaica: A Sexual History of the Jews. Julian Press; 1967. p. 30.

88   Kroh, Rabbi Paysach. *Bris Milah*. ArtScroll, Mesorah Publications Ltd; 2nd edition; https://www.amazon.com/Bris-Milah-Circumcision-compendium-anthologized /dp/0899061974.

89   Panati, Charles. *Sexy Origins and Intimate Things: The Rites and Rituals of Straights, Gays, Bi's, Drags, Trans, Virgins, and Others*. Kindle Edition. 2012. loc. 1365, https:// www.amazon.com/dp/B00AN959CW#detailBullets_feature_div.

90   Kirsch, Adam. *The People and the Books*. Norton; 2016. Loc. 384, https://books
     .google.com/books/about/The_People_and_the_Books.html?id=hMBojw
     EACAAJ.

91   Edwardes, Allen. Erotica Judaica: A Sexual History of the Jews. New York: Julian
     Press; 1967. p. 30.

92   The exception is the last 8 verses of Deuteronomy, describing Moses' death and burial
     that, tradition has it, was written by Joshua.

93   Friedman, Richard Elliot. *Who Wrote the Bible?*, Simon & Schuster; 2019. p. 212.

94   Propp, William. Origins of the Bible, https://www.youtube.com/watch?v=iNH8kP
     h3V5Y.

95   *When Abraham and Sarah traveled to Egypt during a famine, they presented themselves
     as brother and sister rather than as husband and wife. This lead to a case of mistaken
     identity, which was eventually discovered.*

96   *Joseph's brothers came to Egypt during a famine, to buy grain. They did not recognize
     Joseph, who had risen to a position of power in Egypt. Joseph tested his brothers and even-
     tually revealed his true identity to them.*

97   *Moses' mother placed him in a basket and set him afloat on the Nile River to protect him
     from Pharaoh's decree to kill all Hebrew male infants. Pharaoh's daughter discovered the
     baby Moses while bathing in the river, and decided to adopt him as her own son, keeping
     his true identity as a Hebrew child a secret.*

98   Wikipedia. There is no chronological order in the Torah, https://en.wikipedia.org
     /wiki/There_is_no_chronological_order_in_the_Torah.

99   L., Abigail. When Did Abraham Live? *New Creation*. 2023-06-21.

100 Potok, Chaim. *Wanderings*. Knopf; 1978. p. 23, https://books.google.com/books
     /about/Wanderings.html?id=G6htAAAAMAAJ.

101 Roberts, John R. When was Genesis Written? 2021Located at: SIL International.

102 Wright, Jacob. *Why the Bible Began: An Alternative History of Scripture and its
     Origins*. Cambridge University Press; 2023. p. 37, https://www.amazon.com/dp
     /B0C94TGL1H.

103 Hoffman, L. A. *Covenant of Blood: Circumcision and Gender in Rabbinic Judaism*.
     University of Chicago Press; 1996. p. 28. As cited in Fleiss, Endnote 24.

104 Bloom, Harold, Rosenberg, David. *The Book of J*. Grove Press; 2004. p. 9.

105 Cohen, Shaye J. D. *Why aren't Jewish women circumcised? : gender and covenant in
     Judaism*. University of California Press; 2005. p. 9.

106 https://www.scientificamerican.com/article/why-humans-have-no-penis-bone/.

107 Stern, David. *The Jewish Bible: A Material History*. University of Washington Press;
     2017. p. 17.

108 Wolbe, Rabbi Aryeh. An Unbroken Chain of Torah Transmission. Blog, https://
     www.simpletoremember.com/vitals/chain.htm.

109 https://ots.org.il/the-chain-of-torah-transmission-and-its-implications-today/.

110 Freedman, Harry. *The Murderous History of Bible Translations: Power, Conflict, and the
     Quest for Meaning*. 2022. p. 12–15.

111 https://www.google.com/search?q=dead+sea+scrolls&oq=dead+se&aqs=chrome.o
     .oj46l2j69i57j46jol3.1941joj4&sourceid=chrome&ie=UTF-8.

112 Stern, David. *The Jewish Bible: A Material History*. University of Washington Press; 2017. p. 17.

113 Meredith Corp. *The Dead Sea Scrolls*. New York, NY: Meredith Corp.; 2021. p. 26.

114 Propp, William. Origins of the Bible. YouTube, https://www.youtube.com/watch ?v=iNH8kPh3V5Y.

115 Hays, J. Daniel. Reconsidering the Height of Goliath. *JETS*. 2021; 48(4):701–14.

116 Trey-the-explainer. Who is Lilith? Adam's first wife? YouTube, https://www.youtube .com/watch?v=2F90C4cByhA.

117 Klotz, Charles. 1,153 Fun Facts: To Leave You Astounded. 2021. loc. 663.

118 Propp, William. Origins of the Bible, https://www.youtube.com/watch?v=iNH8k Ph3V5Y.

119 Freedman, Harry. *The Murderous History of Bible Translations: Power, Conflict, and the Quest for Meaning*—Kindle edition by Freedman, Harry. Religion & Spirituality Kindle eBooks @ Amazon.com. 2022. p. 12–15.

120 Stern, David. *The Jewish Bible: A Material History*. University of Washington Press; 2017. p. 17.

121 Wikipedia. Jacob ben Chayyim, https://en.wikipedia.org/wiki/Jacob_ben_Hayyim _ibn_Adonijah.

122 Propp, William. Origins of the Bible. YouTube, https://www.youtube.com/watch?v= iNH8kPh3V5Y.

123 Hoffman, L. A. *Covenant of Blood: Circumcision and Gender in Rabbinic Judaism*. University of Chicago Press; 1996. p. 28 Page is unknown. As cited in Fleiss, Endnote 24.

124 Cohen, Shaye J. D. *Why aren't Jewish women circumcised? : gender and covenant in Judaism*. University of California Press; 2005. p. 9.

125 Kirsch, Adam. *The People and the Books*. Norton; 2016. Loc. 384, https://books .google.com/books/about/The_People_and_the_Books.html?id=hMBojwEACAAJ.

126 Gupta, Sujata. Fractured Rituals. *Science News*. 2020; 198(8-15-20):20–25.

127 Frankel, Rabbi David. Joshua Circumcises Israel in Response to Egypt's Scorn. Blog, https://www.thetorah.com/article/joshua-circumcises-israel-in-response-to-egypts -scorn.

128 @JasonFairfield0, https://x.com/JasonFairfield0/status/1746970420857745580.

129 Cohen, Shaye, J. D. Alexander the Great and Jaddus the High Priest According to Josephus. *AJS Review*. 1982–3; 7(8):41–68.

130 Freeman, Phillip. *The Art of Manliness Podcast*. The Audacious Command of Alexander the Great, https://www.artofmanliness.com/articles/alexander-the-great/.

131 Konner, Melvin. *The Jewish Body: An Anatomical History of the Jewish People*. Schocken; 2009. Loc. 537, https://www.amazon.com/dp/B001OLRMU0.

132 Gollaher, David. *Circumcision: A History of the World's most Controversial Surgery*. Basic Books, A Member of the Perseus Books Group; 2000. p. 5.

133 Blanton, Thomas. Philo of Alexandria, Circumcision, and the Construction of the Ethnic "Other" in Greek and Roman Art. Hypotheses. 2021, https://genitaliaandco .hypotheses.org/648.

134 Bigelow, Jim. *The Joy of Uncircumcising!*, 1994. p. 62, https://amazon.com/Joy-Uncircumcising-Circumcision-Psychology-Restoration/dp/093406122X/ref=sr_1_1?dchild=1&keywords=Jim+BIgelow+circumcision&qid=1597452884&sr=8-1.

135 Edwardes, Allen. *Erotica Judaica; A Sexual History of the Jews.* Julian Press; 1967.

136 Friedman, David M. *A Mind of Its Own: A Cultural History of the Penis.* Free Press; 2001. p. 92, https://www.amazon.com/dp/B003719FSM/ref=dp-kindle-redirect?_encoding=UTF8&btkr=1.

137 1 Macc 1:48.

138 2 Macc 6:10.

139 Thiede, Rabbi Barbara. Asking Questions About Circumcision: Is that Allowed? Blog, https://adrenalinedrash.com/?p=2126.

140 Sometimes transliterated as peri'ah, with an apostrophe.

141 Friedman, David M. *A Mind of Its Own: A Cultural History of the Penis.* Free Press; 2001. p. 92, https://www.amazon.com/dp/B003719FSM/ref=dp-kindle-redirect?_encoding=UTF8&btkr=1.

142 Edwardes, Allen. Erotica Judaica: A Sexual History of the Jews. New York: Julian Press; 1967. p. 115.

143 *Mishnah Moed Sabbath 19:6.*

144 Rabbi Eliezer's commentary on Genesis 17, as cited in Glick, p. 52.

145 HaNasi, Rabbi Yehuda. *Mishnah Nedarim 3.*

146 Circumstitions. A Comparison of Intact and Circumcised Penises, http://www.circumstitions.com/Restric/comparison.html.

147 Sprecher, Shlomo. Mezizah Be-Peh—Therapeutic Touch or Hippocratic Vestige? *Hakirah—The Flatbush Journal of Jewish Law and Thought.* 2017; 3.

148 Shabbat 19:3.

149 B. Shabbat 133b.

150 Papa, Rav. *Talmud Shabbat.* 3rd century. p. 133b.

151 Jewishideas.org. Metzitzah B'Peh—Oral Law? https://www.jewishideas.org/article/metzitzah-bpeh-oral-law.

152 Fleiss, Paul, Hodges, Frederick. *What Your Doctor May Not Tell You About Circumcision.* Hachette Book Group; 2002. p. 2.

153 Glick, Leonard B. *Marked in your flesh: circumcision from ancient Judea to modern America.* Oxford: Oxford University Press; 2007. p. 32–33.

154 Toviah Garber, Shemuel. *The Circular Cut: Problematizing the Longevity of Civilization's Most Aggressively Defended Amputation.* Wesleyan University; 2013, https://www.academia.edu/4589882/The_Circular_Cut_Problematizing_the_Longevity_of_Civilization_s_Most_Aggressively_Defended_Amputation.

155 Cooper, Eitan. *Milah Confronts Modernity: Analyzing Debates Over Circumcision Technique.* Brandeis University; 2012. p. 89.

156 Jewishideas.org. Metzitzah B'Peh—Oral Law? https://www.jewishideas.org/article/metzitzah-bpeh-oral-law.

157 Cooper, Eitan. *Milah Confronts Modernity: Analyzing Debates Over Circumcision Technique.* Brandeis University; 2012. p. 89.

158 Cooper, Eitan. *Milah Confronts Modernity: Analyzing Debates Over Circumcision Technique.* Brandeis University; 2012. p. 89.

159 Oster, Marcy. 4 New York City infants have contracted herpes from circumcision rite in past 6 months. *The Jewish World*. The article is no longer available online.

160 Gesundheit, Benjamin, Grisaru-Soen, Galia, Greenberg, David, et al. Neonatal genital herpes simplex virus type 1 infection after Jewish ritual circumcision: modern medicine and religious tradition. *Pediatrics*. 2004; 114(2):e259–e263, https://doi.org/10.1542/peds.114.2.e259.

161 Brady, Brittany. Babies' herpes linked to circumcision practice. CNN, https://www.cnn.com/2013/04/07/health/new-york-neonatal-herpes/index.html.

162 Jensen, K. Thor. New York mohel accused of infecting infant with herpes during circumcision. *Newsweek*. 2019-09-23, https://www.newsweek.com/rabbi-infant-penis-herpes-1460790.

163 Herriman, Robert. Neonatal herpes following ritual circumcision (metzitzah b'peh). *Outbreak News Today*, http://outbreaknewstoday.com/neonatal-herpes-following-ritual-circumcision-metzitzah-bpeh-87323/.

164 Jensen, K. Thor. New York mohel accused of infecting infant with herpes during circumcision. *Newsweek*. 2019-09-23, https://www.newsweek.com/rabbi-infant-penis-herpes-1460790.

165 Orthodox families won't identify circumcisers who gave babies herpes, NYC health spokesman says. Jewish Telegraphic Agency; 2017-04-19, https://www.jta.org/2017/04/19/united-states/orthodox-families-wont-identify-circumcisers-who-gave-babies-herpes-nyc-health-spokesman-says.

166 Romberg, Henry MD. *Bris Milah: A Book About the Jewish Ritual of Circumcision*. Feldheim Publishers; 1982. p. 191.

167 Cooper, Eitan. *Milah Confronts Modernity: Analyzing Debates Over Circumcision Technique*. Brandeis University; 2012. p. 8.

168 Montaigne, Michel De, Trechmann, E. J. *The Diary of Montaigne's Journey to Italy in 1580 and 1581*. 1929. p. 134.

169 Cooper, Eitan. *Milah Confronts Modernity: Analyzing Debates Over Circumcision Technique*. Brandeis University; 2012. p. 89.

170 Kveller Staff. Kveller, https://www.kveller.com/article/the-bris-ceremony/.

171 Glass, J. M. Religious circumcision: a Jewish view. *BJU Int*. 2000; 85(4):560.

172 Epstein, Joseph. Opinion | Pious Agnosticism as a Form of Judaism. *Wall Street Journal*, https://www.wsj.com/articles/mere-pious-agnosticism-jewish-religion-faith-israel-fae3de2d.

173 No to forced circumcision. *Haaretz*. November 29, 2013, https://www.haaretz.com/opinion/no-to-forced-circumcision-1.5295569.

174 StyleLikeU. StyleLikeU Uniforms: The Substance of Hasidic Style. Accessed November 1, 2013. YouTube, https://www.youtube.com/watch?v=ywGhoG3x-50.

175 Israel Story. *Alone Together—Part 1: Mazal Tov!* Israel Story. June 30.

176 Waysman, Dvora. Jewish ritual is the secret to our survival, https://www.jpost.com/jerusalem-report/article-721747.

177 John, Timothy. Jewish Circumcision—What It Was, Is and Can Be. Accessed Feb. 26, 2021. YouTube, https://www.youtube.com/watch?v=YRwPSb6ry70.

178 Pollack, Miriam. Circumcision: Identity, Gender, and Power. *Tikkun*, https://www.tikkun.org/circumcision-identity-gender-and-power.

179 Glick, Leonard B. *Marked in your Flesh: Circumcision from Ancient Judea to Modern America*. Oxford: Oxford University Press; 2007. p. 32–33.

180 Unitarian Universalist Congregation of Phoenix. UUCP Worship Service 2023/06/04—Few Decisions In Life Are Permanent . . . Except Circumcision. YouTube, https://www.youtube.com/watch?v=7Xb2rSn5oZ4.

181 Rebecca Wald, Lisa Braver Moss. *Celebrating Brit Shalom*. First ed. Notim Press; 2014. p. 2.

182 Ungar-Sargon, Eliyahu. Why Is The Reform Movement Scared of Circumcision? March 27, 2018, https://www.eliungar.com/circumcision/2018/3/27/why-is-the -reform-movement-scared-of-circumcision.

183 Goodman, J. Jewish circumcision: an alternative perspective. *Br J Urol*. 1999; 83(1):22–27.

184 Wine, Sherwin. Circumcision. *Humanistic Judaism*. 1998; 16 (Summer 1998):7–8.

185 Bonobo3D. Jewish American Scholar Leonard Glick—Circumcision. YouTube, https://www.youtube.com/watch?v=c4UEbsg-k5Y&list=PLKua sLinBzLvg-s777BUtAX23LTdDfU6g&index=11&t=0s.

186 Ahituv, Netta. Even in Israel, More and More Parents Choose Not to Circumcise Their Sons. *Haaretz*. June 14, 2012, https://www.haaretz.com/even-in-israel-more-and -more-parents-choose-not-to-circumcise-1.5178506.

187 Ungar-Sargon, Eliyahu. Trends in Judaism. Speech given at the Intaction conference held on August 14, 2022 in Atlanta, GA; 2022.

188 *Jewish World*. March 11, 2010. The article is no longer available online.

189 Gradstein, Linda. Circumcision Rates Are Slipping—Even In Israel. *Forward*, https:// forward.com/news/israel/391496/circumcision-rates-are-slipping-even-in-israel/.

190 Rebecca Wald, Lisa Braver Moss. *Celebrating Brit Shalom*. First ed. Notim Press; 2014. p. 2.

191 Rebecca Wald, Lisa Braver Moss. *Celebrating Brit Shalom*. First ed. Notim Press; 2014. p. 2.

192 Ingall, Marjorie. To Cut or Not To Cut: Finding Alternatives to Circumcision. *Tablet Magazine*, http://www.tabletmag.com/jewish-life-and-religion/178356/alternatives -to-circumcision.

193 Moss, Lisa Braver. "Don't Ask, Don't Tell"—Non-circumcising Families in the Jewish Community. YouTube, https://www.youtube.com/watch?v=6_he3TUhTFQ& feature=emb_logo. Jewish Community Center.

194 Silvers, Emma. Brit shalom is catching on, for parents who don't want to circumcise their child. *J The Jewish News of Northern California*. 2012-01-06, https://www.jweekly .com/2012/01/06/alternative-ritual-sans-snip-catching-on-in-bay-area/.

195 Michaelson, Jay. A Modest Proposal. *Forward*. June 27, 2011, https://forward.com /culture/139100/a-modest-proposal/.

196 Cohen-Almagor, Raphael. Should liberal government regulate male circumcision performed in the name of Jewish tradition? *SN Social Sciences*. 2020/11/09; 1(1):20, https://doi.org/10.1007/s43545-020-00011-7.

197 Ben-Yami, Hanoch. Circumcision: What should be done? *J Med Ethics*. 2013; 39(7):459–462, https://doi.org/10.1136/medethics-2012-101274.

198 Goodman, J. Jewish circumcision: an alternative perspective. *Br J Urol*. 1999;
83(1):22–27.

199 The Guardian. Circumcision: 'Penises are a taboo subject' | Modern Masculinity.
YouTube, https://www.youtube.com/watch?v=nSVMgCRI2h8.

200 Center for Countering Digital Hate. *Failure to Protect*. 2021, https://252f2edd-1c8b
-49f5-9bb2-cb57bb47e4ba.filesusr.com/ugd/f4d9b9_08ab7f4e6ef44ff4a05044d
8aef3f3b7.pdf.

201 Global Anti-semitic Attitudes. 2014, https://global100.adl.org/map.

202 Mohammed, Yasmine. *Unveiled: How Western Liberals Empower Radical Islam*. Free
Hearts Free Minds; 2019. p. 52–3.

203 Badiell, David. *Jews Don't Count*. TLS Books; 2021, https://www.amazon.com/dp
/B084GJ78FJ.

204 Kulish, Nicholas. "German Ruling Against Circumcising Boys Draws Criticism". *New
York Times*. June 26, 2012.

205 Toviah Garber, Shemuel. *The Circular Cut: Problematizing the Longevity of
Civilization's Most Aggressively Defended Amputation*. Wesleyan University; 2013,
https://www.academia.edu/4589882/The_Circular_Cut_Problematizing_the
_Longevity_of_Civilization_s_Most_Aggressively_Defended_Amputation.

206 Knobloch, Charlotte. Wollt ihr uns Juden noch? *Süddeutschen Zeitung*. Sept. 25, 2012.

207 Eddy, Melissa. Accord sought in Germany over circumcision issue. *New York Times*.
Aug. 21, 2012.

208 Jordan, Austin. The Cruelty of Circumcision. *Ethican Magazine*. 2019-12-01. Article
has been deleted online.

209 Samuels, Shimon. Does an International Campaign to Ban Brit Mila Contribute to
Antisemitism? *The Jerusalem Post*, https://www.jpost.com/opinion/does-an
-international-campaign-to-ban-brit-mila-contribute-to-antisemitism-629796.

210 Beyond the, Bris. Standing Against Antisemitism, https://www.beyondthebris.com
/standing-against-antisemitism/.

211 Hebblethwaite, Cordelia. Circumcision, the Ultimate Parenting Dilemma. *BBC News
Magazine*. 20 Aug 2012, https://www.bbc.com/news/magazine-19072761.

212 Van Howe, R. S. *Sexual Mutilations: A Human Tragedy*. 1997. Loc. 2879, https://www
.amazon.com/Sexual-Mutilations-Tragedy-Defense-Research-ebook/dp/B000SEP
E8Q/ref=sr_1_9?dchild=1&keywords=marilyn+milos&qid=1598373261&sr=8-9.

213 Stein, D. H., Schroeder, J., Hobson, N. M., Gino, F., Norton, M. I. When alterations
are violations: Moral outrage and punishment in response to (even minor) alterations
to rituals. *J Pers Soc Psychol*. Jan 25, 2021; https://doi.org/10.1037/pspi0000352.

214 UNAIDS, Joint United Nations Programme on HIV/AIDS. 2012. Neonatal and
child male circumcision: a global review (World Health Organization) (2012).

215 Wikipedia. Prevalence of circumcision, https://en.wikipedia.org/wiki/Prevalence
_of_circumcision#cite_note-WHO-25.

216 Wikipedia. Prevalence of circumcision, https://en.wikipedia.org/wiki/Prevalence
_of_circumcision#cite_note-WHO-25.

217 Anwer, Abdul Wahid, Samad, Lubna, Iftikhar, Sundus, Baig-Ansari, Naila. Reported
Male Circumcision Practices in a Muslim-Majority Setting. *Biomed Res Int*.
2017:4957348, https://doi.org/10.1155/2017/4957348.

218 Zaynab El Bernoussi, Baudoin Dupret. Circumcision. *HAL Open Science*. May 26, 2020.

219 Susan Terkel, Lorna Greenberg. *The Circumcision Decision: An Unbiased Guide for Parents*. Carrot Seed Publishing LLC; 2012. loc. 302.

220 Friedman, David M. *A Mind of Its Own: A Cultural History of the Penis*. Free Press; 2001. p. 92, https://www.amazon.com/dp/B003719FSM/ref=dp-kindle-redirect?_encoding=UTF8&btkr=1.

221 Zaynab El Bernoussi, Baudoin Dupret. Circumcision. *HAL Open Science*. May 26, 2020.

222 D'Agati, Mauro. Ouch Ouch Ouch Ouch Ouch! *Vice*. Sept. 1, 2007. Article has been deleted online.

223 Zaynab El Bernoussi, Baudoin Dupret. Circumcision. *HAL Open Science*. May 26, 2020.

224 @Bloodstainedmen, https://x.com/BloodstainedMen/status/1746994051721875739.

225 Meddings, Jonathan. *The Final Cut: The truth about circumcision*. 2022. p. 105, https://www.amazon.com/Final-Cut-truth-about-circumcision/dp/0645368202/ref=sr_1_1?crid=1I3QHKoOIRK4M&keywords=the+final+cut+circumcision&qid=1702883041&s=books&sprefix=the+final+cut+circumcision%2Cstripbooks%2C121&sr=1-1.

226 Wikipedia. Criticism of hadith, https://en.wikipedia.org/wiki/Criticism_of_hadith.

227 Amin, Mohammed. How reliable are Hadith? Some are contradictory, February 14, 2015. Blog, https://www.mohammedamin.com/Community_issues/How-reliable-are-hadith.html#:~:text=Some%20Muslims%20regard%20all%20hadith,that%20hadith%20vary%20in%20reliability.

228 Kamali, Mohammad Hashim. *A Textbook of Hadith Studies: Authenticity, Compilation, Classification and Criticism of Hadith*. 2014, https://www.amazon.com/Textbook-Hadith-Studies-Authenticity-Classification-ebook/dp/B00H6UZUS4/ref=tmm_kin_swatch_0?_encoding=UTF8&qid=&sr=.

229 Gollaher, David. *Circumcision: A History of the World's most Controversial Surgery*. Basic Books, A Member of the Perseus Books Group; 2000. p. 5.

230 Bertaux-Navoiseau, Michel. *The Koran Forbids Circumcision and Excision (updated 02.08.2023)*. 2020, https://www.researchgate.net/publication/344058577_The_Koran_forbids_circumcision_and_excision_updated_02082023.

231 el-Sharkawy, Youssra. Egyptian anti-circumcision group calls for an end to 'male genital mutilation'. *Al-Monitor*. 2019-12-11, https://www.al-monitor.com/pulse/originals/2019/12/egyptians-dispute-necessity-of-circumcision.html.

232 Rosen, Michael. Anesthesia for ritual circumcision in neonates. *Paediatr Anaesth*. 2010; 20(12):1124–1127, https://doi.org/10.1111/j.1460-9592.2010.03445.x.

233 Zaynab El Bernoussi, Baudoin Dupret. Circumcision. *HAL Open Science*. May 26, 2020.

234 Amin, Mohammed. Review of "A Textbook of Hadith Studies: Authenticity, Compilation, Classification and Criticism of Hadith" by Mohammad Hashim Kamali. 2023, https://www.mohammedamin.com/Reviews/A-Textbook-of-Hadith-Studies.html.

235 Abu-Sahlieh, S. A. To Mutilate in the Name of Jehovah or Allah: Legitimization of Male and Female Circumcision. *Med Law*. 1994; 13(7–8):575–622. Complete article not available.

236 To Mutilate in the Name of Jehovah or Allah: Legitimization of Male and Female Circumcision. *Med Law*. July 1994 1994; 13(7–8):575–622.

237 Cumhur, M. Ethical evaluation of non-therapeutic male circumcision. *Turkish Journal of Psychiatry*. 2014.

238 Zaynab El Bernoussi, Baudoin Dupret. Circumcision. *HAL Open Science*. May 26, 2020.

239 Bertaux-Navoiseau, Michel. *The Koran forbids circumcision and excision* (updated 02/08/2023). 2020, https://www.researchgate.net/publication/344058577_The_Koran_forbids_circumcision_and_excision_updated_02082023.

240 Kelley, Debbie. Bloodstained Men and other groups' push to not circumcise infant boys seen as anti-Semitic by some, a child-protection issue by others. *The Gazette*. 2022-02-12, https://gazette.com/news/local/bloodstained-men-and-other-groups-push-to-not-circumcise-infant-boys-seen-as-anti-semitic/article_9dbd6e82-89cd-11ec-8484-3350f6acc8e7.html.

241 Susan Terkel, Lorna Greenberg. *The Circumcision Decision: An Unbiased Guide for Parents*. Carrot Seed Publishing LLC; 2012. loc. 302, https://www.amazon.com/Circumcision-Decision-Unbiased-Guide-Parents-ebook/dp/B00BAVEEOG/ref=sr_1_1?crid=2J82MDF76IWX2&keywords=the+circumcision+decision&qid=1648087022&sprefix=%2Caps%2C235&sr=8-1.

242 Meddings, Jonathan. *The Final Cut: The truth about circumcision*. 2022. p. 105, https://www.amazon.com/Final-Cut-truth-about-circumcision/dp/0645368202/ref=sr_1_1?crid=1I3QHK0OIRK4M&keywords=the+final+cut+circumcision&qid=1702883041&s=books&sprefix=the+final+cut+circumcision%2Cstripbooks%2C121&sr=1-1.

243 https://en.wikipedia.org/wiki/Religious_male_circumcision.

244 Fr. Clark, Peter A. To Circumcise or Not to Circumcise? *Journal of the Catholic Health Association of the United States*. 2006; September-October.

245 The Catholic Church. Catechism of The Catholic Church, https://www.usccb.org/sites/default/files/flipbooks/catechism/II/.

246 United States Conference of Catholic Bishops. *Ethical and Religious Directives for Catholic Health Care Services*. 2009:29.

247 Darby, Robert. *A Surgical Temptation: The Demonization of the Foreskin and the Rise of Circumcision in Britain eBook: Darby, Robert: Kindle Store*. University of Chicago Press; 2013. p. 4.

248 *Benedict XVI General Audience*. Retrieved from http://w2.vatican.va/content/benedict-xvi/en/audiences/2007/documents/hf_ben-xvi_aud_20070131.html. January 2007.

249 Fr. Clark, Peter A. To Circumcise or Not to Circumcise? *Journal of the Catholic Health Association of the United States*. 2006; September-October.

250 Staff, Catholic Answers. The Catechism forbids deliberate mutilation, so why is non-therapeutic circumcision allowed? *Catholic Answers*, https://www.catholic.com/qa/the-catechism-forbids-deliberate-mutilation-so-why-is-non-therapeutic-circumcision-allowed.

251 Popcak, Greg. Mating Matters. Podcast. Feb. 20, 2019.

252 Cox G, Morris B. J. *Why Circumcision: From Prehistory to the Twenty-First Century* | *SpringerLink*. SpringerLink; 2012, https://link.springer.com/chapter/10.1007/978-1 -4471-2858-8_21#citeas.

253 Winchester, Simon. *Knowing What We Know: The Transmission of Knowledge: From Ancient Wisdom to Modern Magic*. Harper; 2023. p. 27.

254 Schoen, Edgar. Circumcision is not only Jewish, its good for you. *J the Jewish Weekly of Northern California*. 2013-01-04.

255 Kepler, Dawn. My daughter won't circumcise her son—what can I do? *J the Jewish Weekly of Northern California*. 2018-11-02.

256 Kepler, Dawn. Circumcision still a volatile topic—can divide be breached? *J the Jewish Weekly of Northern California*. 2020-01-24.

257 Laqueur, Thomas. *Solitary Sex: A Cultural History of Masturbation*. Zone Books; 2003, https://amazon.com/dp-1890951323/dp/1890951323/ref=mt_hardcover?_ encoding=UTF8&me=&qid=1591800744.

258 Milos, M. F., Kirkwood, Judy. *Please Don't Cut the Baby: A Nurse's Memoir*. loc. 784.

259 Darby, Robert. *A Surgical Temptation: The Demonization of the Foreskin and the Rise of Circumcision in Britain*. University of Chicago Press; 2013. p. 4.

260 Darby, Robert. *A Surgical Temptation: The Demonization of the Foreskin and the Rise of Circumcision in Britain*. University of Chicago Press; 2013. p. 3.

261 When I was a child, the cereal was called Kellogg's Sugar Frosted Flakes, in later years Kellogg dropped the word "Sugar." Kellogg's Frosted Flakes are banned in all of Europe and Japan because they contain BHT.

262 Friedman, David M. *A Mind of Its Own: A Cultural History of the Penis*. Free Press; 2001. p. 92, https://www.amazon.com/dp/B003719FSM/ref=dp-kindle-redirect? _encoding=UTF8&btkr=1.

263 Markel, Howard. Were Kellogg's Corn Flakes Created as an 'Anti-Masturbatory Morning Meal'? https://www.snopes.com/fact-check/kelloggs-corn-flakes -masturbation/.

264 Graham, Sylvester. *A Lecture to Young Men on Chastity*. 1834.

265 Scott, Joe. 5 Reasons The Victorian Era Was Utter Insanity | Answers With Joe. YouTube, https://www.youtube.com/watch?v=3IDN9gTAtjg.

266 Tinari, Paul. *Lymph Mobbed & Booby Trapped: How Modern Culture, the Fashion Industry and Politicized Medicine Conspire to Keep Women Sick and How YOU Can Get Healthy Again*. 2017, https://www.amazon.com/dp/B06WRV7XGW.

267 Thanks to Kellogg I ate the nutritionally deficient Kellogg's Sugar Frosted Flakes for many boyhood breakfasts.

268 Goldman, Ronald. *Circumcision, The Hidden Trauma: How an American Cultural Practice Affects Infants and Ultimately Us All*. Vanguard; 1997. p. 58.

269 Kellogg, John Harvey. Plain Facts for Old and Young, https://en.wikipedia.org/wiki /John_Harvey_Kellogg#cite_note-plainfacts-37.

270 Chubak, Barbara. 1101 The Orthopedic Origin of Popular Male Circumcision in America. *Journal of Urology*. 2013; 189(4S):e451-e451, https://doi.org/doi:10.1016/j .juro.2013.02.693.

271 Panati, Charles. *Sexy Origins and Intimate Things: The Rites and Rituals of Straights, Gays, Bi's, Drags, Trans, Virgins, and Others*. Kindle Edition. 2012. loc. 1365, https://www.amazon.com/dp/B00AN959CW#detailBullets_feature_div.

272 Darby, Robert. Book Review by Robert Darby. 2002, https://web.archive.org/web/20080719031737/http:/www.circinfo.org/review.html.

273 Leckie, Robert. *Helmet for My Pillow: From Parris Island to the Pacific*. Arcadia Press; 2019. p. 2, https://www.amazon.com/dp/B07S91DQ1N.

274 Bloom, Howard. *How I Accidentally Started The Sixties*. Rare Bird Books, A Vireo Book (September 12, 2017); 2017. loc. 4393, https://www.amazon.com/dp/B075FR2JCS.

275 Guest, Christopher. A Historical and Medical Critique of Circumcision. https://www.youtube.com/watch?v=XwZiQyFaAso&list=PLKuasLinBzLvg-s777BUtAX23LTdDfU6g&index=39&t=0s.

276 Remondino, P. Negro rapes and their social problems. *National Popular Review—1894* Jan 4(1): 3–6. 1894.

277 Ritter, Thomas J. *Say No to Circumcision!: 40 Compelling Reasons Why You Should Respect His Birthright and Keep Your Son Whole*. 2020. p. 11–12.

278 Darby, Robert. *A Surgical Temptation: The Demonization of the Foreskin and the Rise of Circumcision in Britain*. University of Chicago Press; 2013. p. 3.

279 Friedman, David M. *A Mind of Its Own: A Cultural History of the Penis*. Free Press; 2001. p. 92, https://www.amazon.com/dp/B003719FSM/ref=dp-kindle-redirect?_encoding=UTF8&btkr=1.

280 Wolbarst, Abraham L. Universal Circumcision as a Sanitary Measure. *JAMA*. 1914:92–97.

281 Guest, Christopher. A Historical and Medical Critique of Circumcision. Accessed March 25, 2016, https://www.youtube.com/watch?v=XwZiQyFaAso&list=PLKuasLinBzLvg-s777BUtAX23LTdDfU6g&index=39&t=0s.

282 Wiswell, T. E., Smith, F. R., Bass, J. W. Decreased incidence of urinary tract infections in circumcised male infants. *Pediatrics*. May 1985; 75(5):901–3.

283 Bailey, Robert C., Egesah, Omar, Rosenberg, Stephanie. Male circumcision for HIV prevention: a prospective study of complications in clinical and traditional settings in Bungoma, Kenya. *Bull World Health Organ*. 2008; 86(9):669–677, https://doi.org/10.2471/blt.08.05148.

284 Bobrow, Emily. The industrialized world is turning against circumcision. It's time for the US to consider doing the same. *Quartz*. Jan. 17, 2017, https://qz.com/885018/why-is-circumcision-so-popular-in-the-us/.

285 Gairdner, D. The fate of the foreskin, a study of circumcision. *Br Med J*. Dec 24 1949; 2(4642):1433–7, https://doi.org/10.1136/bmj.2.4642.1433.

286 Oster, J. Further fate of the foreskin. Incidence of preputial adhesions, phimosis, and smegma among Danish schoolboys. *Arch Dis Child*. Apr 1968; 43(228):200–203, https://doi.org/10.1136/adc.43.228.200.

287 Ko, M. C., Liu, C. K., Lee, W. K., Jeng, H. S., Chiang, H. S., Li, C. Y. Age-specific prevalence rates of phimosis and circumcision in Taiwanese boys. *J Formos Med Assoc*. Apr 2007; 106(4):302–7, https://doi.org/10.1016/s0929-6646(09)60256-4.

288 Abhinav Agarwal, Anup Mohta Ritesh K. Anand. Preputial Retraction in Children. *Journal of Indian Association of Pediatric Surgeons*. 2005; 10(2):89–91.

289 Thorvaldsen, M. A., Meyhoff, H. H. Patologisk eller fysiologisk fimose? [Pathological or physiological phimosis?]. *Ugeskr Laeger*. Apr 25, 2005; 167(17):1858–62.

290 Abhinav Agarwal, Anup Mohta Ritesh K. Anand. Preputial Retraction in Children. *Journal of Indian Association of Pediatric Surgeons*. 2005; 10(2):89–91.

291 Denniston, George C., Hill, George. Gairdner was wrong. *Can Fam Physician*. 2010; 56(10):986–987.

292 Riddle, D. L., Jiranek, W. A., Hayes, C. W. Use of a validated algorithm to judge the appropriateness of total knee arthroplasty in the United States: a multicenter longitudinal cohort study. *Arthritis Rheumatol*. Aug 2014; 66(8):2134–43, https://doi.org /10.1002/art.38685.

293 Dekker, Rebecca. *Babies Are Not Pizzas: They're Born, Not Delivered*. Evidence Based Birth: 2019. p. 101, https://www.amazon.com/gp/product/B07WQGZ695/ref=ppx _yo_dt_b_search_asin_title?ie=UTF8&psc=1.

294 Theoharakis, Matthew, NewYork-Presbyterian Morgan Stanley Children's Hospital, New York N. Y., Feldman, Evin, et al. Circumcision. *Pediatrics In Review*. 2024; 43(12):728–730, https://doi.org/10.1542/pir.2022-005536.

295 Chamberlain, David B. Babies Remember Pain. *Pre and Perinatal Psychology*. 1989; 3(4):297–310.

296 CIRP. cirp.org. article no longer available online

297 Wan, Julian. Gomco Circumcision Clamp: An Enduring and Unexpected Success. *Urology*. 2002; 59:790–791.

298 Yarbrough, Danielle. *1,500 Fascinating Facts*. Amazon Publishing. loc. 523, https:// www.amazon.com/dp/B08P13HZML.

299 Losquadro, Anthony. Dr. Health Radio Fast Moving Discussion on Circumcision. The Circumcision Chronicles Uncut Podcast. 2019.

300 Burd, Eileen M., Dean, Christina L. Human Papillomavirus. *Microbiol Spectr*. 2016; 4(4):10.1128/microbiolspec.DMIH2-0001-2015, https://doi.org/10.1128/microbiol spec.DMIH2-0001-2015.

301 Manini, I., Montomoli, E. Epidemiology and prevention of Human Papillomavirus. *Ann Ig*. Jul-Aug 2018; 30(4 Supple 1):28–32, https://doi.org/10.7416/ai.2018.2231.

302 Sabeena, Sasidharanpillai, Bhat, Parvati, Kamath, Veena, Arunkumar, Govindakarnavar. Possible non-sexual modes of transmission of human papilloma virus. *J Obstet Gynaecol Res*. 2017; 43(3):429–435, https://doi.org/10.1111/jog.13248.

303 HPV-16,-18, -31, -33, -35, -39, -45, -51, -52, -56, -58, -59, -66, -68, -82.

304 Manini, I., Montomoli, E. Epidemiology and prevention of Human Papillomavirus. *Ann Ig*. Jul-Aug 2018; 30(4 Supple 1):28–32, https://doi.org/10.7416/ai.2018.2231.

305 Mobini Kesheh, M., Keyvani, H. The Prevalence of HPV Genotypes in Iranian Population: An Update. *Iran J Pathol*. Summer 2019; 14(3):197–205, https://doi.org /10.30699/ijp.2019.90356.1861.

306 Auvert, Bertran, et al. Randomized, controlled intervention trial of male circumcision for reduction of HIV infection risk: the ANRS 1265 Trial. *PLoS Med*. 2005; 2(11):e298-e298, https://doi.org/10.1371/journal.pmed.0020298.

307 Huang, Liang-Liang, et al. Circumcision reduces the incidence of human papillomavirus infection in men. *Zhonghua Nan Ke Xue*. 2018; 24(4):327–330.

308 Manini, I., Montomoli, E. Epidemiology and prevention of Human Papillomavirus. *Ann Ig.* Jul-Aug 2018; 30(4 Supple 1):28–32, https://doi.org/10.7416/ai.2018.2231.

309 Pahud, Barbara A., Ault, Kevin A. The Expanded Impact of Human Papillomavirus Vaccine. *Infect Dis Clin North Am.* 2015; 29(4):715–724, https://doi.org/10.1016/j.idc.2015.07.007.

310 Petrosky, E., Bocchini, J. A., Jr., Hariri, S., et al. Use of 9-valent human papillomavirus (HPV) vaccine: updated HPV vaccination recommendations of the advisory committee on immunization practices. *MMWR Morb Mortal Wkly Rep.* Mar 27, 2015; 64(11):300–304.

311 Centers for Disease Control and Prevention. Vaccinating Boys and Girls Against HPV | CDC. 2020.

312 SciShow. Why HPV Is Cancer In One Convenient Package. YouTube, https://www.youtube.com/watch?v=xNJgf9Z5v4M.

313 Cunningham, Aimee. HPV tests could replace Pap smears. *Science News.* August 4, 2018:9.

314 Bailey, Robert C., Moses, Stephen, Parker, Corette B., et al. Male circumcision for HIV prevention in young men in Kisumu, Kenya: a randomised controlled trial. *The Lancet.* 2007/02/24; 369(9562):643–656, https://doi.org/10.1016/S0140-6736(07)60312-2.

315 Auvert, B., Taljaard, D., Lagarde, E., Sobngwi-Tambekou, J., Sitta, R., Puren, A. Randomized, controlled intervention trial of male circumcision for reduction of HIV infection risk: the ANRS 1265 Trial. *PLoS Med.* Nov 2005; 2(11):e298, https://doi.org/10.1371/journal.pmed.0020298.

316 Gray, R. H., Kigozi, G., Serwadda, D., et al. Male circumcision for HIV prevention in men in Rakai, Uganda: a randomised trial. *Lancet.* Feb 24, 2007; 369(9562):657–66, https://doi.org/10.1016/s0140-6736(07)60313-4.

317 Riess, Thomas H., Achieng', Maryline M., Otieno, Samuel, Ndinya-Achola, J. O., Bailey, Robert C. "When I Was Circumcised I Was Taught Certain Things": Risk Compensation and Protective Sexual Behavior among Circumcised Men in Kisumu, Kenya. *PLoS One.* 2010; 5(8):e12366, https://doi.org/10.1371/journal.pone.0012366.

318 Gisselquist, David, Wilkinson, Robert. *Points to Consider: Responses to HIV/AIDS in Africa, Asia, and the Caribbean.* 2020, https://www.researchgate.net/publication/311743040_Points_to_Consider_Responses_to_HIVAIDS_in_Africa_Asia_and_the_Caribbean_By_David_Gisselquist_London_Adonis_Abbey_2008_223_pp_illustrated_7900_hardcover.

319 Van Howe, R. S. The Fragility Index in HIV/AIDS Trials. *J Gen Intern Med.* Jul 2020; 35(7):2204, https://doi.org/10.1007/s11606-019-05554-x.

320 Mills, E., Siegfried, N. Cautious optimism for new HIV/AIDS prevention strategies. *Lancet.* Oct 7, 2006; 368(9543):1236, https://doi.org/10.1016/s0140-6736(06)69513-5.

321 Fox, Maggie. Circumcision helps protect men, not women from AIDS. 2009-07-17.

322 Lei, Jun hao, Liu, Liang ren, Wei, Qiang, et al. Circumcision Status and Risk of HIV Acquisition during Heterosexual Intercourse for Both Males and Females: A Meta-Analysis. *PLoS One.* 2015; https://doi.org/10.1371/journal.pone.0125436.

323 Gray, R. H., Kigozi, G., Serwadda, D., et al. Male circumcision for HIV prevention in men in Rakai, Uganda: a randomised trial. *Lancet.* Feb 24, 2007; 369(9562):657–66, https://doi.org/10.1016/s0140-6736(07)60313-4.

324 Jones, Ryan. *Crucial Dissent Went Unreported—Circumcision Stakeholders in Africa*. Feb. 8, 2021, https://www.foregen.org/commentarium-articles/circumcision -stakeholders-in-africa.

325 Perera, Caryn L., et al. Safety and efficacy of nontherapeutic male circumcision: a systematic review. *Ann Fam Med*. Jan-Feb 2010; 8(1):64–72, https://doi.org/10.1370 /afm.1073.

326 Glick, Leonard B. *Marked in your flesh : circumcision from ancient Judea to modern America*. Oxford: Oxford University Press; 2007. p. 32–33.

327 Garenne, M. Long-term population effect of male circumcision in generalised HIV epidemics in sub-Saharan Africa. *Afr J AIDS Res*. May 2008; 7(1):1–8, https://doi.org /10.2989/ajar.2008.7.1.1.429.

328 Darby, Robert, Van Howe, Robert. Not a surgical vaccine: there is no case for boosting infant male circumcision to combat heterosexual transmission of HIV in Australia. *Australian and New Zealand Journal of Public Health*. 2011; 35(5).

329 Shahvisi, Arianne, Tangwa, Godfrey, Earp, Brian. A new Tuskegee? Unethical human experimentation and Western neocolonialism in the mass circumcision of African men. *Developing World Bioethics*. 2020/09/11:in press, https://doi.org/10.1111/dewb .12285.

330 Sidler, D, Smith, J, Rode, H. Neonatal circumcision does not reduce HIV/AIDS infection rates. *SAMJ: South African Medical Journal*. 2008; 98:762–766.

331 Erickson, John A. Does Male Circumcision Help Spread AIDS? http://www.sexually mutilatedchild.org/does-c.htm.

332 Nayan, M., Hamilton, R. J., Juurlink, D. N., Austin, P. C., Jarvi, K. A. Circumcision and Risk of HIV Among Males From Ontario, Canada. *J Urol*. Sep 23, 2021; https:// doi.org/10.1097/ju.0000000000002234.

333 Frisch, Morten, Simonsen, Jacob. Non-therapeutic male circumcision in infancy or childhood and risk of human immunodeficiency virus and other sexually transmitted infections: national cohort study in Denmark. *European Journal of Epidemiology*. 2021/09/26; https://doi.org/10.1007/s10654-021-00809-6.

334 Kenyon, C. R., Vu, L., Menten, J., Maughan-Brown, B. Male circumcision and sexual risk behaviors may contribute to considerable ethnic disparities in HIV prevalence in Kenya: an ecological analysis. *PLoS One*. 2014; 9(8):e106230, https://doi.org/10.1371 /journal.pone.0106230.

335 Reynolds, S. J., Shepherd, M. E., Risbud, A. R., et al. Male circumcision and risk of HIV-1 and other sexually transmitted infections in India. *Lancet*. Mar 27, 2004; 363(9414):1039–40, https://doi.org/10.1016/s0140-6736(04)15840-6.

336 Centers for Disease Control and Prevention. 2017. HIV (@CDCgov) (2017).

337 Mbugua, G. G., et al. Epidemiology of HIV infection among long distance truck drivers in Kenya. *East Afr Med J*. Aug 1995; 72(8):515–8.

338 Glick, Leonard B. *Marked in your flesh : circumcision from ancient Judea to modern America*. Oxford: Oxford University Press; 2007. p. 32–33.

339 Reuters Health. Circumcision may not curb gay HIV transmission. 2010-12-07, https://www.reuters.com/article/business/healthcare-pharmaceuticals/circumcision -may-not-curb-gay-hiv-transmission-idUSTRE6B65W3/.

340 Hart, Lisa M. McDaid, Helen, A. Weiss, Graham, J. Circumcision among men who have sex with men in Scotland: limited potential for HIV prevention. 2010-10-01; https://doi.org/10.1136/sti.2010.042895.

341 Medpagetoday. Circumcision May Be Protective Against HIV in Men Who Have Sex With Men. 2023-07-20, https://www.medpagetoday.com/meetingcoverage/ias /105561.

342 Gray, R. H., Wawer, M. J., Brookmeyer, R., et al. Probability of HIV-1 transmission per coital act in monogamous, heterosexual, HIV-1-discordant couples in Rakai, Uganda. *Lancet*. Apr 14, 2001; 357(9263):1149–53, https://doi.org/10.1016/s0140 -6736(00)04331-2.

343 UNAIDS, Joint United Nations Programme on HIV/AIDS. 2012. Neonatal and child male circumcision: a global review (World Health Organization) (2012).

344 UNAIDS and WHO. 2019. Voluntary Medical Male Circumcision Rising (2019).

345 Helen Clark, et al. A future for the world's children? A WHO–UNICEF–Lancet Commission—The Lancet. *The Lancet*. 2020; 395(10224):605–658, https://doi.org /doi:10.1016/S0140-6736(19)32540-1.

346 Earp, Brian. Between Moral Relativism and Moral Hypocrisy: Reframing the Debate on "FGM." *Kennedy Inst Ethics J*. 2016/07/28; 26:105–144, https://doi.org/10.1353 /ken.2016.0009.

347 Earp, Brian David. May 11, 2021, https://x.com/briandavidearp/status/13922956212523 70433.

348 Samuelson, Julia. Voluntary Medical Male Circumcision in an Evolving HIV Prevention Landscape in East and Southern Africa. presented at: 20th International Conference on AIDS and STIs in Africa; 2019; Session What's New: HIV Prevention, https://hivpreventioncoalition.unaids.org/en/resources/voluntary-medical-male -circumcision-evolving-hiv-prevention-landscape-east-and-southern.

349 Rosenberg, Molly S., Gómez-Olivé, Francesc X., Rohr, Julia K., Kahn, Kathleen, Bärnighausen, Till W. Are circumcised men safer sex partners? Findings from the HAALSI cohort in rural South Africa. *PLoS One*. 2018; 13(8):e0201445, https://doi .org/10.1371/journal.pone.0201445.

350 Keetile, Mpho. An assessment of sexual risk behaviours among circumcised and uncircumcised men before and after the implementation of the safe male circumcision programme in Botswana. *AIDS Care*. 2020:1–8, https://doi.org/10.1080/09540121.20 20.1769830.

351 Bonobo3D. Male Circumcision & HIV, https://www.youtube.com/watch?v=RGdA-P1YWYjo&list=PLKuasLinBzLvg-s777BUtAX23LTdDfU6g&index=14&t=0s.

352 Moodley, Jayajothi, Naidoo, Sarita, Kelly, Cliff, Reddy, Tarylee, Ramjee, Gita. The Impact of Male Partner Circumcision on Women's Health Outcomes. *AIDS Education and Prevention*. 2020/08/01; 32(4):356–366, https://doi.org/10.1521/aeap .2020.32.4.356.

353 Hines, J. Z., Sachathep, K., Pals, S., et al. HIV incidence by male circumcision status from the population-based HIV impact assessment (PHIA) surveys-eight sub-Saharan African countries, 2015–2017. *J Acquir Immune Defic Syndr*. Mar 16, 2021; https://doi.org/10.1097/qai.0000000000002658.

354 Adams, Alfred, Moyer, Eileen. Sex is never the same: men's perspectives on refusing circumcision from an in-depth qualitative study in Kwaluseni, Swaziland. *Glob Public Health*. 2015; 10(5–6):721–738, https://doi.org/10.1080/17441692.2015.1004356.

355 Peck, Megan E., et al. HIV, syphilis, and hepatitis B virus infection and male circumcision in five Sub-Saharan African countries: Findings from the Population-based HIV Impact Assessment surveys, 2015–2019 | PLOS Global Public Health. 2023; https://doi.org/10.1371/journal.pgph.0002326.

356 Bailey, Robert C., Egesah, Omar, Rosenberg, Stephanie. Male circumcision for HIV prevention: a prospective study of complications in clinical and traditional settings in Bungoma, Kenya. *Bull World Health Organ*. 2008; 86(9):669–677, https://doi.org/10.2471/blt.08.051482.

357 https://icap.columbia.edu/cpt_projects/volunteer-medical-male-circumcision-vmmc/.

358 https://www.facebook.com/IntactKenya/.

359 US Preventive Services Task Force. Preexposure Prophylaxis for the Prevention of HIV Infection: US Preventive Services Task Force Recommendation Statement. *JAMA*. 2019; 321(22):2203–2213, https://doi.org/10.1001/jama.2019.6390.

360 Kaldor, John M., Wilson, David P. How low can you go: the impact of a modestly effective HIV vaccine compared with male circumcision. *AIDS*. 2010; 24(16):2573–2578, https://doi.org/10.1097/QAD.0b013e32833ead96.

361 Kaldor, John M., Wilson, David P. How low can you go: the impact of a modestly effective HIV vaccine compared with male circumcision. *AIDS*. 2010; 24(16):2573–2578, https://doi.org/10.1097/QAD.0b013e32833ead96.

362 Stephenson, Kathryn E., Wagh, Kshitij, Korber, Bette, Barouch, Dan H. Vaccines and Broadly Neutralizing Antibodies for HIV-1 Prevention. *Annual Review of Immunology*. 2020; 38(1):673–703, https://doi.org/10.1146/annurev-immunol-080219-023629.

363 Liu, Angus. Watch out, GSK. Gilead's twice-yearly PrEP drug shows 100% efficacy for HIV prevention. *Fierce Pharma*. 2024/06/20, https://www.fiercepharma.com/pharma/watch-out-gsk-gileads-twice-yearly-prep-drug-shows-100-efficacy-hiv-prevention.

364 Ark Invest. FYI podcast. Using Gene Editing to Cure HIV with Daniel Dornbusch, https://www.youtube.com/watch?v=FcgbIJHVL-A.

365 Smith, G. L., Greenup, R., Takafuji, E. T. Circumcision as a risk factor for urethritis in racial groups. *American journal of public health*. 1987; 77(4):452–454, https://doi.org/10.2105/ajph.77.4.452.

366 Donovan, Basil, Bassett, I., Bodsworth, Neil. Male circumcision and common sexually transmissible diseases in a developed nation setting. *Genitourinary medicine*. 11/01 1994; 70:317–20, https://doi.org/10.1136/sti.70.5.317.

367 Bassett, I., Donovan, B., Bodsworth, N. J., et al. Herpes simplex virus type 2 infection of heterosexual men attending a sexual health centre. *Med J Aust*. Jun 6 1994; 160(11):697–700.

368 Frisch, Morten, Simonsen, Jacob. Non-therapeutic male circumcision in infancy or childhood and risk of human immunodeficiency virus and other sexually transmitted infections: national cohort study in Denmark. *European Journal of Epidemiology*. 2021/09/26; https://doi.org/10.1007/s10654-021-00809-6.

369 Hooykaas C, van der Velde FW, van der Linden MM. et al.. The importance of ethnicity as a risk factor for STDs and sexual behaviour among heterosexuals. *Genitourin Med*. 1991. 67(5):378–83.

370 Michael, R. T., Wadsworth, J., Feinleib, J., Johnson, A. M., Laumann, E. O., Wellings, K. Private sexual behavior, public opinion, and public health policy related to sexually transmitted diseases: a US-British comparison. *American journal of public health*. 1998; 88(5):749–754, https://doi.org/10.2105/ajph.88.5.749.

371 Boyle, G. J., Goldman, R., Svoboda, J. S., Fernandez, E. Male circumcision: pain, trauma and psychosexual sequelae. *J Health Psychol*. May 2002; 7(3):329–43, https://doi.org/10.1177/135910530200700310.

372 onlinedoctor. Prevalence of STDs Across the United States and Europe, https://onlinedoctor.superdrug.com/std-us-eu.html.

373 American Academy of Family Physicians. Neonatal Circumcision. @aafp blog, https://www.aafp.org/about/policies/all/neonatal-circumcision.html.

374 Morris, Brian J., Gray, Ronald H., Castellsague, Xavier, et al. The Strong Protective Effect of Circumcision against Cancer of the Penis. *Adv Urol*. 2011:812368, https://doi.org/10.1155/2011/812368.

375 American Society of Clinical Oncology. Penile Cancer: Risk Factors and Prevention, https://www.cancer.net/cancer-types/penile-cancer/risk-factors-and-prevention.

376 Us Department of Commerce, Noaa National Weather Service. *How Dangerous is Lightning?* 2019. March 12th 2019 4:22 AM, https://www.weather.gov/safety/lightning-odds.

377 Frisch, Morten, Aigrain, Yves, et al. Cultural Bias in the AAP's 2012 Technical Report and Policy Statement on Male Circumcision. *Pediatrics*. 2013; 131(4):796–800, https://doi.org/10.1542/peds.2012-2896.

378 Guest, Christopher. A Historical and Medical Critique of Circumcision / Intact Babies: Avoiding Clinical Errors. https://www.youtube.com/watch?v=Ya4K5K_ESOg.

379 Schmidt, Bogdana, Copp, Hillary L. Work-up of Pediatric Urinary Tract Infection. *Urol Clin North Am*. 2015; 42(4):519–526, https://doi.org/10.1016/j.ucl.2015.05.011.

380 Knight, J. F. Urinary Tract Infection. *Current Opinion in Pediatrics*. 1991; 3:43.

381 Wiswell, T. E., Smith, F. R., Bass, J. W. Decreased incidence of urinary tract infections in circumcised male infants. *Pediatrics*. May 1985; 75(5):901–3.

382 Thompson, H. C., King, L. R., Knox, E., Korones, S. B. Report of the ad hoc task force on circumcision. *Pediatrics*. Oct 1975; 56(4):610–11.

383 Chessare, J. B. Circumcision: is the risk of urinary tract infection really the pivotal issue? *Clin Pediatr (Phila)*. Feb 1992; 31(2):100–104, https://doi.org/10.1177/000992289203100207.

384 Amato, Dante Garduno-Espinosa Juan. Circumcision of the Newborn Male and the risk of Urinary Tract Infection During the First Year: A Meta-Analysis. *Boletino Medico Infante Mexico*. 1992; 49(10):652–658.

385 Baskin, Laurence. Neonatal circumcision: Risks and benefits. *UpToDate*. Jan 2024.

386 Amir, J., Varsano, I., Mimouni, M. Circumcision and urinary tract infection in infants. *Am J Dis Child*. Nov 1986; 140(11):1092.

387 Hoffman, Thomas. Male circumcision greatly increases risk of urinary tract problems. *sciencenordiccom*. 2016-12-30.

388 Fleiss, Paul, Hodges, Frederick. *What Your Doctor May Not Tell You About Circumcision*. Hachette Book Group; 2002. p. 2.

389 Frisch, Morten, Aigrain, Yves, et al. Cultural Bias in the AAP's 2012 Technical Report and Policy Statement on Male Circumcision. *Pediatrics*. 2013; 131(4):796–800, https://doi.org/10.1542/peds.2012-2896.

390 Chessare, J. B. Circumcision: is the risk of urinary tract infection really the pivotal issue? *Clin Pediatr (Phila)*. Feb 1992; 31(2):100–104, https://doi.org/10.1177/000992 289203100207.

391 Goldman, M., Barr, J., Bistritzer, T., Aladjem, M. Urinary tract infection following ritual Jewish circumcision. *Isr J Med Sci*. 1996; 32(11):1098–1102.

392 Prais, D., Shoov-Furman, R., Amir, J. Is ritual circumcision a risk factor for neonatal urinary tract infections? *Arch Dis Child*. 2009; 94(3):191–194, https://doi.org/10.1136/adc.2008.144063.

393 Toker, Ori, Schwartz, Shepard, Segal, Gershon, Godovitch, Nadia, Schlesinger, Yechiel, Raveh, David. A costly covenant: ritual circumcision and urinary tract infection. *Isr Med Assoc J*. 2010; 12(5):262–265.

394 Cohen, H. A., Drucker, M. M., Vainer, S., et al. Postcircumcision urinary tract infection. *Clin Pediatr (Phila)*. Jun 1992; 31(6):322–324, https://doi.org/10.1177/00099 2289203100601.

395 Horwitz, Jonathan, Schussheim, Arnold, Scalettar, Howard E. Abdominal Distension Following Ritual Circumcision. *Pediatrics*. 1976; 57(4):579.

396 Eason, J. D., McDonnell, M., Clark, G. Male ritual circumcision resulting in acute renal failure. *BMJ*. Sep 10 1994; 309(6955):660–61, https://doi.org/10.1136/bmj.309.6955.660.

397 Personal Communication with Dr. M. Hakim. 2024.

398 Brown, Mark S., Brown, Cheryl A. Circumcision Decision: Prominence of Social Concerns. *Pediatrics*. 1987; 80(2):215–219.

399 Scott, Kellie. Should we circumcise our son just because his dad is? *ABC Everyday*. 2021-03-22, https://www.abc.net.au/everyday/should-we-circumcise-our-son-just-because-his-dad-is/100012216.

400 Bigelow, Jim. The Joy of Uncircumcising. 2nd ed. Kearney NE: Morris Publishing; 2002. p. 33.

401 Bigelow, Jim. The Joy of Uncircumcising. 2nd ed. Kearney NE: Morris Publishing; 2002. p. 26–27.

402 Narvaez, Darcia. Doctor Ignorance of Male Anatomy Harms Boys. 2011, http://www.psychologytoday.com/blog/moral-landscapes/201110/doctor-ignorance-male-anatomy-harms-boys.

403 Sneppen, Ida, Thorup, Jørgen. Foreskin Morbidity in Uncircumcised Males. *Pediatrics*. 2016:e20154340, https://doi.org/10.1542/peds.2015-4340.

404 Frisch, Morten, Earp, Brian D. Circumcision of male infants and children as a public health measure in developed countries: A critical assessment of recent evidence. *Glob Public Health*. 2018/05/04; 13(5):626–641, https://doi.org/10.1080/17441692.2016.11 84292.

405 Shankar, K. R., Rickwood, A. M. The incidence of phimosis in boys. *BJU Int.* 1999; 84(1):101–102, https://doi.org/10.1046/j.1464-410x.1999.00147.x.

406 Wallerstein, Edward. *Circumcision: An American Health Fallacy.* 1980. p. 128, https://www.amazon.com/Circumcision-American-Health-Fallacy-SPRINGER/dp/0826132413.

407 Bollinger, Dan. The Penis-Care Information Gap: Preventing Improper Care of Intact Boys. *Thymos: Journal of Boyhood Studies.* 2007/07/01; 1:205–219, https://doi.org/10.3149/thy.0205.219.

408 Iwamuro, S., Furuta, A., Iwanaga, S., et al. Foreskin retraction for phimosis of the newborn. *Nihon Hinyokika Gakkai Zasshi.* Jan 1997; 88(1):35–9, https://doi.org/10.5980/jpnjurol1989.88.35.

409 Ball, Peter. A Survey of Subjective Foreskin Sensation in 600 Intact Men. In: Denniston G. C. HFM, Milos M. F., ed. *Bodily integrity and the Politics of Circumcision.* 2012.

410 Mathew, Vivin Thomas Varghese, Abraham. Evaluating the role of topical steroids as a primary intervention for treatment of phimosis in pediatric age group. Original Research Articles. *International Surgery Journal.* 2020-10-23; 7(11), https://www.ijsurgery.com/index.php/isj/article/view/6689.

411 Rendy, Andika, Rodjani, Arry, Wahyudi, Irfan. Efficacy of topical steroid therapy for phimosis treatment: a systematic review. Circumcision, phimosis, topical steroid. *2020.* 2020-03-05; 11(1):5, https://doi.org/10.15562/ism.v11i1.633.

412 Steadman, B., Ellsworth, P. To circ or not to circ: indications, risks, and alternatives to circumcision in the pediatric population with phimosis. *Urol Nurs.* Jun 2006; 26(3):181–94. https://pubmed.ncbi.nlm.nih.gov/16800325/.

413 Ashfield, J. E., Nickel, K. R., Siemens, D. R., MacNeily, A. E., Nickel, J. C. Treatment of phimosis with topical steroids in 194 children. *J Urol.* Mar 2003; 169(3):1106–8, https://doi.org/10.1097/01.ju.0000048973.26072.eb.

414 Schultheiss, D., Truss, M. C., Stief, C. G., Jonas, U. Uncircumcision: a historical review of preputial restoration. *Plast Reconstr Surg.* 1998; 101(7):1990–1998, https://doi.org/10.1097/00006534-199806000-00037.

415 phimostop.com. PhimoStop™: the leader in non-surgical phimosis treatment, https://www.phimostop.com/en/.

416 Chung, E., AndroUrology, Centre, Polikarpov, D., et al. (080) Psychological Outcomes and Sexual Satisfaction Rates in Males with Phimosis Following the Novoglan Foreskin Extender Treatment. *J Sex Med.* 2024; 21(Supplement_2), https://doi.org/10.1093/jsxmed/qdae002.072.

417 Hotonu, Sesi, Mohamed, Ahmed, Rajimwale, Ashok, Gopal, Milan. Save the foreskin: Outcomes of preputioplasty in the treatment of childhood phimosis. *The Surgeon.* 2020/06/01/; 18(3):150–153, https://doi.org/10.1016/j.surge.2019.08.004.

418 Nunn, Gary. "I have phimosis, a condition that makes it painful to pull back the foreskin. After my brother's death, I learned he also had it." *Insider.* 2023-07-13, https://www.insider.com/brothers-with-phimosis-painful-foreskin-2023-7.

419 Kidger, E. A., Haider, N., Qazi, A. Acquired phimosis after plastibell circumcision: a preventable consequence. *Ann R Coll Surg Engl.* 2012; 94(6):e186-e188.

420 Gulin, Sandra Jerkovic, Lundin, Filippa, Seifert, Oliver. Comorbidity in patients with Lichen sclerosus: a retrospective cohort study. Original Paper. *European Journal of Medical Research*. 2023-09-11; 28(1):1–8, https://doi.org/doi:10.1186/s40001-023-01335-9.

421 Jayakumar, S., Antao, B., Bevington, O., Furness, P., Ninan, G. K. Balanitis xerotica obliterans in children and its incidence under the age of 5 years. *J Pediatr Urol*. Jun 2012; 8(3):272–5, https://doi.org/10.1016/j.jpurol.2011.05.001.

422 Lowry-Lehnen, Theresa. Lichen sclerosus: An overview. *The Medical Independent*. October 8, 2023.

423 Lander, Mervyn. *Sexual Mutilations: A Human Tragedy*. 1997. Loc. 2227, https://www.amazon.com/Sexual-Mutilations-Tragedy-Defense-Research-ebook/dp/B000SEPE8Q/ref=sr_1_9?dchild=1&keywords=marilyn+milos&qid=1598373261&sr=8-9.

424 Navarrete, Jorge, Echarte, Lourdes, Sujanov, Alexandra, et al. Platelet-rich plasma for male genital lichen sclerosus resistant to conventional therapy: first prospective study. *Dermatologic Therapy*. (n/a):e14032, https://doi.org/10.1111/dth.14032.

425 Milos, Marilyn. Do You Know . . . About Yeast Infections?—Intact America. 2021, https://intactamerica.org/dyk_yeast-infections/.

426 Chivers, Chloe. Men's Sexual Wellness: Education Drives Empowerment. *Men's Sexual Wellness: Educational Empowerment* blog. 2024, https://kolorex.co.nz/blogs/blog/men-s-sexual-wellness-education-drives-empowerment.

427 Wallerstein, Edward. *Circumcision: An American Health Fallacy*. 1980. p. 128, https://www.amazon.com/Circumcision-American-Health-Fallacy-SPRINGER/dp/0826132413.

428 Romberg, Henry MD. *Bris Milah: A Book About the Jewish Ritual of Circumcision*. Feldheim Publishers; 1982. p. 191.

429 Sherman, M., Sherman, I. C. Sensori-motor responses in infants. *Journal of Comparative Psychology*. 1925; 5(1):53–68, https://doi.org/10.1037/h0074472.

430 Anand, K. J., Hickey, P. R. Pain and its effects in the human neonate and fetus. *N Engl J Med*. Nov 19 1987; 317(21):1321–9, https://doi.org/10.1056/nejm198711193172105.

431 Goksan, Sezgi, Hartley, Caroline, Emery, Faith, et al. fMRI reveals neural activity overlap between adult and infant pain. *eLife*. 2015/04/21; 4:e06356, https://doi.org/10.7554/eLife.06356.

432 Some typical scales are NIPS, Children's Hospital Eastern Ontario Pain Scale, the Faces Pain Scale-Revised and FLACC (Face, Legs, Activity, Cry, Consolability).

433 Boyle, G. J., Goldman, R., Svoboda, J. S., Fernandez, E. Male circumcision: pain, trauma and psychosexual sequelae. *J Health Psychol*. May 2002; 7(3):329–43, https://doi.org/10.1177/13591053020070310.

434 Howard, Cynthia Howard Fred Weitzman Michael. Acetaminophen Analgesia In Neonatal Circumcision. *Pediatrics*. 1994-04-30; 93(4):641–646.

435 Ryan, C. A., Finer, N. N. Changing attitudes and practices regarding local analgesia for newborn circumcision. *Pediatrics*. Aug 1994; 94(2 Pt 1):230–33.

436 Williamson, P. S., Williamson, M. L. Physiologic stress reduction by a local anesthetic during newborn circumcision. *Pediatrics*. Jan 1983; 71(1):36–40.

437 Stang, Howard J., Gunnar, Megan R., Snellman, Leonard, Condon, Lawrence M., Kestenbaum, Roberta. Local Anesthesia for Neonatal Circumcision: Effects on

Distress and Cortisol Response. *JAMA*. 1988; 259(10):1507–1511, https://doi.org/10
.1001/jama.1988.03720100025033.

438 Fleiss, P. M. Letters. *The Lancet*. 1995; 345:927.

439 Fleiss, Paul, Hodges, Frederick. *What Your Doctor May Not Tell You About Circumcision*. Hachette Book Group; 2002. p. 2.

440 Lander, J., Brady-Fryer, B., Metcalfe, J. B., Nazarali, S., Muttitt, S. Comparison of ring block, dorsal penile nerve block, and topical anesthesia for neonatal circumcision: a randomized controlled trial. *Jama*. Dec 24–31 1997; 278(24):2157–62.

441 Goldstein, Pavel, Weissman-Fogel, Irit, Dumas, Guillaume, Shamay-Tsoory, Simone G. Brain-to-brain coupling during handholding is associated with pain reduction. *Proceedings of the National Academy of Sciences*. 2018; 115(11):E2528-E2537, https://doi .org/10.1073/pnas.1703643115.

442 Gunnar, M. R., Connors, J., Isensee, J., Wall, L. Adrenocortical activity and behavioral distress in human newborns. *Dev Psychobiol*. May 1988; 21(4):297–310, https://doi.org /10.1002/dev.420210402.

443 Romberg, Rosemary. Circumcision: The Painful Dilemma. 2nd ed. Bergin & Garvey Publishers; 1985:p. vii.

444 Romberg, Rosemary. Circumcision: The Painful Dilemma. 2nd ed. Bergin & Garvey Publishers; 1985:p. 321.

445 Bellieni, Carlo V. Neonatal Infant Pain Scale in assessing pain and pain relief for newborn male circumcision. *International Journal of Impotence Research*. 2022/03/29; https://doi.org/10.1038/s41443-022-00551-x.

446 Chamberlain, David. cirp.org, http://www.cirp.org/library/psych/chamberlain/.

447 Taddio, A., Goldbach, M., Ipp, M., Stevens, B., Koren, G. Effect of neonatal circumcision on pain responses during vaccination in boys. *Lancet*. Feb 4 1995; 345(8945):291–2, https://doi.org/10.1016/s0140-6736(95)90278-3.

448 Page, Gayle Giboney. Are There Long-Term Consequences of Pain in Newborn or Very Young Infants? *The Journal of Perinatal Education*. 2004; 13(3)(2004 Summer):10–17, https://doi.org/10.1624%2F105812404X1725.

449 Fitzgerald, M., Beggs, S. The neurobiology of pain: developmental aspects. *Neuroscientist*. Jun 2001; 7(3):246–57, https://doi.org/10.1177/107385840100700309.

450 Fu, Xin, Teboul, Eric, Weiss, Grant L., et al. Gq neuromodulation of BLA parvalbumin interneurons induces burst firing and mediates fear-associated network and behavioral state transition in mice. *Nature Communications*. 2022/03/11; 13(1):1290, https://doi.org/10.1038/s41467-022-28928-y.

451 ScienceDaily. Study examines why the memory of fear is seared into our brains. 2022; https://www.sciencedaily.com/releases/2022/06/220601133030.htm.

452 Fleiss, Paul, Hodges, Frederick. *What Your Doctor May Not Tell You About Circumcision*. Hachette Book Group; 2002. p. 2.

453 Margulis, Jennifer. *The Business of Baby*. Scribner, A Division of Simon & Schuster, Inc.; 2013. p. 133.

454 Rabinowitz, Ronald, Hulbert, William C. Newborn Circumcision Should Not Be Performed Without Anesthesia. *Birth*. 1995; 22(1):45–46, https://doi.org/10.1111 /j.1523-536X.1995.tb00554.x

455 Taylor, H. Does lidocaine-prilocaine cream (EMLA) decrease the pain of neonatal circumcision? *Am Fam Physician*. Feb 15, 2004; 69(4):909–10.

456 http://www.thewholenetwork.org/twn-news/infant-circumcision-with-anesthesia -does-it-really-help-the-pain.

457 Modekwe, Victor Ifeanyichukwu, Ugwu, Jideofor Okechukwu, Ekwunife, Okechukwu Hyginus, et al. A Randomised Controlled Trial on the Efficacy and Safety of Oral Ketamine in Neonatal Circumcision. *Journal of Clinical & Diagnostic Research*. 2021; 15(1):1–4.

458 Roshan Chanchlani, Shabeeh Nazar, Gurunath Chavan, Jain, Somya. Paediatric Circumcision with Intravenous (IV) Ketamine, and Penile Block as a Day Care Surgery. 2021; https://doi.org/10.21088/nijs.0976.4747.9118.10.

459 Wanxia WANG, Hong MA, Jin CHEN,Kang CHENG,Meiyu. LIU. Effect of different doses of esketamine combined with sevoflurane anesthesia in pediatric day foreskin surgery. *The Journal of Practical Medicine*. 2024-04-25; 40(8):1078–1082, https://doi.org/10.3969/j.issn.1006-5725.2024.08.010.

460 Ozen, V., Yigit, D. A Comparison of the Postoperative Analgesic Effectiveness of Ultrasound-Guided Dorsal Penile Nerve Block and Ultrasound-Guided Pudendal Nerve Block in Circumcision. *Urol Int*. 2020; https://doi.org/10.1159/000509173.

461 Zadrazil, Markus, Feigl, Georg, Opfermann, Philipp, Marhofer, Peter, Marhofer, Daniela, Schmid, Werner. Ultrasound-Guided Dorsal Penile Nerve Block in Children: An Anatomical-Based Observational Study of a New Anesthesia Technique. *Children*. 2024; 11(1):50.

462 Personal communication with Jeffery Levy, MD.

463 Umami, Andan Firmansyah, Henri, Setiawan, Daniel Akbar, Wibowo, Tita, Rohita, Afriza. Virtual Reality (VR) Media Distraction Relieve Anxiety Level of the Children During Circumcision. presented at: 1st Paris Van Java International Seminar on Health, Economics, Social Science and Humanities; 2021/03/08; Paris, https://www .atlantis-press.com/proceedings/pvj-ishessh-20/125953827.

464 SmileyScope. Smileyscope—Reimagine healthcare. Blog, https://www.smileyscope .com.au/.

465 Willyard, Cassandra. The pain is real. The painkillers are virtual reality. MIT Technology Review. 2023; https://www.technologyreview.com/2023/11/17/1083586 /the-pain-is-real-the-painkillers-are-virtual-reality/.

466 Taddio, A., Pollock, N., Gilbert-MacLeod, C., Ohlsson, K., Koren, G. Combined analgesia and local anesthesia to minimize pain during circumcision. *Arch Pediatr Adolesc Med*. 2000; 154(6):620–623, https://doi.org/10.1001/archpedi.154.6.620.

467 John, Timothy. Nurses of St Vincent: Saying NO to Circumcision (1994). YouTube, https://www.youtube.com/watch?v=Csaal-MqXB4. online.

468 Losquadro, Anthony. Dr. Health Radio Fast Moving Discussion on Circumcision. The Circumcision Chronicles Uncut Podcast, 2019.

469 Lander, J., Brady-Fryer, B., Metcalfe, J. B., Nazarali, S., Muttitt, S. Comparison of ring block, dorsal penile nerve block, and topical anesthesia for neonatal circumcision: a randomized controlled trial. *Jama*. Dec 24–31 1997; 278(24):2157–62.

470 Margulis, Jennifer. *The Business of Baby*. Scribner, A Division of Simon & Schuster, Inc.; 2013. p. 133.

471 Personal communication with Jeffery Levy, MD. 2021.

472 Personal Communication with Jeffrey Levy, MD. 2021.

473 Stang, H. J., Snellman, L. W. Circumcision practice patterns in the United States. *Pediatrics*. Jun 1998; 101(6):E5, https://doi.org/10.1542/peds.101.6.e5.

474 Personal Communication with James Snyder, MD. 2021.

475 John, Timothy. Nurses of St Vincent: Saying NO to Circumcision (1994). YouTube, https://www.youtube.com/watch?v=Csaal-MqXB4. online.

476 Roberts, Jeffrey. Is Male Circumcision A Violation of Human Rights? *Collective Evolution*, https://www.collective-evolution.com/2020/02/13/is-male-circumcision -a-violation-of-human-rights/.

477 National Research Council. *Guide for the Care and Use of Laboratory Animals*. 2020, https://grants.nih.gov/grants/olaw/guide-for-the-care-and-use-of-laboratory-animals .pdf.

478 Ritter, Thomas J. *Say No to Circumcision!: 40 Compelling Reasons Why You Should Respect His Birthright and Keep Your Son Whole*. 2020. p. 11–12.

479 Van Howe, R. S. *Sexual Mutilations: A Human Tragedy*. 1997. Loc. 2879, https://www .amazon.com/Sexual-Mutilations-Tragedy-Defense-Research-ebook/dp/B000SEP E8Q/ref=sr_1_9?dchild=1&keywords=marilyn+milos&qid=1598373261&sr=8-9.

480 Van Howe, R. S. Anaesthesia for Circumcision. 1999; https://doi.org/10.1007/978 -0-585-39937-9_7.

481 Rossi, Serena, Buonocore, Giuseppe, Bellieni, Carlo Valerio. Management of pain in newborn circumcision: a systematic review. *European Journal of Pediatrics*. 2020/08/03; https://doi.org/10.1007/s00431-020-03758-6.

482 Ritter, Thomas J. *Say No to Circumcision!: 40 Compelling Reasons Why You Should Respect His Birthright and Keep Your Son Whole*. 2020. p. 11–12.

483 Cooper, Eitan. *Milah Confronts Modernity: Analyzing Debates Over Circumcision Technique*. Brandeis University; 2012. p. 89.

484 Centers for Disease Control and Prevention. *Information for providers counseling male patients and parents regarding male circumcision and the prevention of HIV infection, STIs, and other health outcomes*. Pamphlet (or booklet). 2018. 22/2018, https://stacks .cdc.gov/view/cdc/58456.

485 Banieghbal, B. Optimal time for neonatal circumcision: An observation-based study. *Journal of Pediatric Urology*. 2009; 5(5):359–362, https://doi.org/10.1016/j.jpurol .2009.01.002.

486 Frisch, Morten, Earp, Brian D. Circumcision of male infants and children as a public health measure in developed countries: A critical assessment of recent evidence. *Glob Public Health*. 2018/05/04; 13(5):626–641, https://doi.org/10.1080/17441692.2016.11 84292.

487 Centers for Disease Control and Prevention. *Information for providers counseling male patients and parents regarding male circumcision and the prevention of HIV infection, STIs, and other health outcomes*. Pamphlet (or booklet). 22/2018, https://stacks.cdc .gov/view/cdc/58456.

488 Pediatrics, American Academy of. Prevention and Management of Procedural Pain in the Neonate: An Update. *Pediatrics*. 2016; 137(2):e20154271, https://doi.org/10.1542 /peds.2015-4271.

489 Zbar, Ross I. S. *Floating Feathers: A Doctor's Harrowing Experience as a Patient Within Conventional Medicine—and an Impassioned Call for the Future of Care in America.* Miles Trevor Press; 2021. loc. 1847, https://amazon.com/Floating-Feathers-Experience-Conventional-Impassioned-ebook/dp/B086WN9TKZ/ref=sr_1_1?dchild=1&key words=zbar%2C+ross&qid=1624979116&sr=8-1.

490 Bonobo3D. Psychiatrist Discusses the Lasting Trauma of Circumcision, https://www.youtube.com/watch?v=117vEwBtEY4&list=PLKuasLinBzLvg-s777BUtAX23LTdDfU6g&index=10&t=0s.

491 Oprah Winfrey & Dr. Bruce Perry in Conversation | SXSW EDU 2021. YouTube, https://www.youtube.com/watch?v=uUAL8RVvkyY&t=81s.

492 Levy, DM. Psychic trauma of operations in children. 1945; 69: 7–25. *Am J Dis Child.* 1945; 69:7–25.

493 Nicole Victoria, Anne Murphy. Exposure to Early Life Pain: Long Term Consequences and Contributing Mechanisms. *Curr Opin Behav Sci.* 2015; https://doi.org/10.1016/j.cobeha.2015.11.015.

494 Miani, Alessandro, et al. Neonatal male circumcision is associated with altered adult socio-affective processing: Heliyon. *Heliyon.* 2020; 6(11), https://doi.org/doi:10.1016/j.heliyon.2020.e05566.

495 Boyle, Gregory J., Ramos, Samuel. Post-traumatic stress disorder (PTSD) among Filipino boys subjected to non-therapeutic ritual or medical surgical procedures: A retrospective cohort study. *Ann Med Surg (Lond).* 2019; 42:19–22, https://doi.org/10.1016/j.amsu.2019.04.004.

496 Ramos, Samule Boyle Gregory. Ritual and Medical Circumcision among Filipino Boys | SpringerLink. In: Denniston G. C. HFM, Milos M. F., ed. *Understanding Circumcision.* SpringerLink; 2020.

497 National Institutes of Health. A Growing Epidemic. *NIH Medline Plus*, https://magazine.medlineplus.gov/pdf/MLP_Winter_09.pdf.

498 Cansever, G. Psychological effects of circumcision. *Br J Med Psychol.* Dec 1965; 38(4):321–31, https://doi.org/10.1111/j.2044-8341.1965.tb01314.x.

499 Bollinger, Dan. Adverse Childhood Experiences, Dysfunctional Households, and Circumcision. *Journal for Prenatal and Perinatal Psychology and Health 36(3), Fall 2022* 2022/12/07; 36(Fall 2022)(3).

500 Tinari, Paul D. Circumcision Permanently Alters the Brain. *Circumcision Resource Center.* 2023.

501 Goldman, Ronald. *Circumcision, The Hidden Trauma : How an American Cultural Practice Affects Infants and Ultimately Us All.* Vanguard; 1997. p. 110.

502 Chamberlain, David. Babies Remember Pain. *Kindred.* Jan. 19, 2016, https://www.kindredmedia.org/2016/01/babies-remember-pain/.

503 Patel, H. The problem of routine circumcision. *Can Med Assoc J.* 1966; 95(11):576–581.

504 Thorup, Jørgen, Thorup, Sebastian Cortes, Ifaoui, Inge Botker Rasmussen. Complication rate after circumcision in a paediatric surgical setting should not be neglected. *Dan Med J.* 2013; 60(8):A4681-A4681.

505 Schröder, Annette, Farhat, Walid A., Chiasson, David, Wilson, Gregory J., Koyle, Martin A. Serious and Fatal Complications after Neonatal Circumcision. *European Urology Focus.* 2022/09/01; 8(5):1560–1563, https://doi.org/10.1016/j.euf.2021.12.005.

506 Manley, Alex. Everything You Need to Know About Circumcision. Feb. 27, 2022.

507 McAllister, Ryan. Child Circumcision: An Elephant in the Hospital. YouTube, https://www.youtube.com/watch?v=Ceht-3xu84I.

508 Ahituv, Netta. Even in Israel, More and More Parents Choose Not to Circumcise Their Sons. *Haaretz*. June 14, 2012, https://www.haaretz.com/even-in-israel-more-and -more-parents-choose-not-to-circumcise-1.5178506.

509 Frisch, Morten, Earp, Brian D. Circumcision of male infants and children as a public health measure in developed countries: A critical assessment of recent evidence. *Glob Public Health*. 2018/05/04; 13(5):626–641, https://doi.org/10.1080/17441692.2016.11 84292.

510 Weiss, Helen A., Larke, Natasha, Halperin, Daniel, Schenker, Inon. Complications of circumcision in male neonates, infants and children: a systematic review. *BMC Urol*. 2010; 10:2–2, https://doi.org/10.1186/1471-2490-10-2.

511 Pieretti-Vanmarcke, Rafael V. Pieretti, Allan, M. Goldstein, Rafael. Late complica-tions of newborn circumcision: a common and avoidable problem. *Pediatric Surgery International*. 2010-02-14; 26(5):515–518, https://doi.org/doi:10.1007/s00383 -010-2566-9.

512 DeMaria, J., Abdulla, A., Pemberton, J., Raees, A., Braga, L. H. Are Physicians Performing Neonatal Circumcisions Well Trained? *Canadian Urological Association Journal*. 2013/08/19; 7(7–8):260–64, https://doi.org/10.5489/cuaj.200.

513 Bonobo3D. Doctor Denounces Circumcision of Children. YouTube, https://www .youtube.com/watch?v=xgGeOvSgPu4.

514 CNBC. How Ultraviolet Light Could Help Stop The Spread of Coronavirus. 2020/05/10, https://www.cnbc.com/2020/05/10/how-ultraviolet-light-could-help -stop-the-spread-of-covid-19.html.

515 Enzenauer, R. W., Dotson, C. R., Leonard, T., Reuben, L., Bass, J. W., Brown, J., 3rd. Male predominance in persistent staphylococcal colonization and infection of the newborn. *Hawaii Med J*. Oct 1985; 44(10):389–90, 392, 394–6.

516 Rabin, R. Rabin R. Mysterious Crop of Staph: Newborns, moms infected after stay at St. Catherine's. *Newsday*, https://www.qcc.cuny.edu/socialSciences/ppecorino/SS640 /READING-Staph-infect-babies.html.

517 Van Howe, R. S., Robson, W. L. The possible role of circumcision in newborn outbreaks of community-associated methicillin-resistant Staphylococcus aureus. *Clin Pediatr (Phila)*. May 2007; 46(4):356–8, https://doi.org/10.1177/0009922806294847.

518 Woodside, J. R. Necrotizing fasciitis after neonatal circumcision. *Am J Dis Child*. 1980; 134(3):301–302, https://doi.org/10.1001/archpedi.1980.02130150055015.

519 Willinger, M., James, L. S., Catz, C. Defining the sudden infant death syndrome (SIDS): deliberations of an expert panel convened by the National Institute of Child Health and Human Development. *Pediatr Pathol*. Sep-Oct 1991; 11(5):677–84, https://doi.org/10.3109/15513819109065465.

520 Elhaik, E. A "Wear and Tear" Hypothesis to Explain Sudden Infant Death Syndrome. *Front Neurol*. 2016; 7:180, https://doi.org/10.3389/fneur.2016.00180.

521 Elhaik, E. Neonatal circumcision and prematurity are associated with sudden infant death syndrome (SIDS). *J Clin Transl Res*. Jan 10, 2019; 4(2):136–151.

522 Goodman, J. Jewish circumcision: an alternative perspective. *Br J Urol.* 1999; 83(1):22–27.

523 Fleiss, Paul, Hodges, Frederick. *What Your Doctor May Not Tell You About Circumcision.* Hachette Book Group; 2002. p. 2.

524 Gairdner, D. The fate of the foreskin, a study of circumcision. *Br Med J.* 1949; 2(4642):1433–1437, https://doi.org/10.1136/bmj.2.4642.1433.

525 American Academy of Pediatrics Task Force on Circumcision. Circumcision policy statement. *Pediatrics.* 2012; 130(3):585–586, https://doi.org/10.1542/peds.2012-1989.

526 HS, Yellen. Bloodless circumcision of the newborn. *Am J Obstet Gynecol.* July 1935; 30(1):146–147.

527 Akman, Mustafa. Is it Reliable to Make a Decision Based on Visual Changes in the Patient's Diaper in the Evaluation of Post-Circumcision Bleeding. *African Journal of Paediatric Surgery.* 2023; https://journals.lww.com/ajps/fulltext/2023/20010/is_it _reliable_to_make_a_decision_based_on_visual.4.aspx.

528 Personal communication with Dr. James Snyder.

529 Rosner, Fred. Hemophilia in the Talmud and Rabbinic Writings. *Annals of Internal Medicine.* 1969; 70(4):833–837.

530 Margulis, Jennifer. *The Business of Baby.* Scribner, A Division of Simon & Schuster, Inc.; 2013. p. 133.

531 Bissada, Nabil K., Morcos, Rafik R., El-Senoussi, Mohamed. Post-Circumcision Carcinoma of the Penis. I. Clinical Aspects. *J Urol.* 1986/02/01/ 1986; 135(2):283–285, https://doi.org/10.1016/S0022-5347(17)45614-X.

532 Cardoso, Thaís, et al. Traumatic neuroma of the penis after circumcision—Case report. *Anais brasileiros de dermatologia.* 2015/05/01; 90:397–9, https://doi.org/10 .1590/abd1806-4841.20153233.

533 Dixon, S., Snyder, J., Holve, R., Bromberger, P. Behavioral effects of circumcision with and without anesthesia. *J Dev Behav Pediatr.* Oct 1984; 5(5):246–50.

534 Marshall, R. E., et al. Circumcision: II. Effects upon mother-infant interaction. *Early Hum Dev.* Dec 1982; 7(4):367–74, https://doi.org/10.1016/0378-3782(82)90038-x.

535 Tan, April, et al. The Effect of Early Circumcision on Breastfeeding Duration Using Sibling Comparisons. *Pediatrics.* 2023; 144(2_MeetingAbstract):273–273, https://doi .org/10.1542/peds.144.2MA3.273.

536 O'Callahan, Cliff, Te, Silena, Husain, Aaftab, Rosener, Stephanie E., Hussain, Naveed. The Effect of Circumcision on Exclusive Breastfeeding, Phototherapy, and Hospital Length of Stay in Term Breastfed Newborns. *Hospital Pediatrics.* 2020:hpeds.2019– 0270, https://doi.org/10.1542/hpeds.2019-0270.

537 Stanford Medicine. Complications of Circumcision. 2023, https://med.stanford.edu /newborns/professional-education/circumcision/complications.html.

538 Fleiss, Paul, Hodges, Frederick. *What Your Doctor May Not Tell You About Circumcision.* Hachette Book Group; 2002. p. 2.

539 Benchekroun, A., Lakrissa, A., Tazi, A., Hafa, D., Ouazzani, N. Fistules uréthrales après circoncision: à propos de 15 cas. [Urethral fistulas after circumcision: Apropos of 15 cases]. *Maroc Med.* Jun-Oct 1981; 3():715–8.

540 Ahmed Zaki Anwar, et al. A three-step repair of post circumcision coronal fistula: A glans flap, urethral closure, and dartos flap interposition. *Journal of Pediatric Surgery*. 2021; 0(0), https://doi.org/10.1016/j.jpedsurg.2020.09.012.

541 Chukwubuike, Kevin. Dorsal Urethrocutaneous Fistula Resulting From Circumcision: Report of a Rare Anomaly. 2021/04/28, https://www.researchgate.net/publication/351184584_Dorsal_Urethrocutaneous_Fistula_Resulting_From_Circumcision_Report_of_a_Rare_Anomaly.

542 Fleiss, Paul, Hodges, Frederick. *What Your Doctor May Not Tell You About Circumcision*. Hachette Book Group; 2002. p. 2.

543 Michael P. Kurtz, Caleb P. Nelson. Urology Mythbusters: Are topical corticosteroids effective for treating postcircumcision penile adhesions? *Journal of Pediatric Urology*. 2020:222–226, https://doi.org/10.1016/j.jpurol.2020.02.007.

544 Tempark, Therdpong, Wu, Tim, Singer, Craig, Shwayder, Tor. Dermatological complications of circumcision: lesson learned from cases in a pediatric dermatology practice. *Pediatr Dermatol*. Sep-Oct 2013; 30(5):519–528, https://doi.org/10.1111/pde.12140.

545 Cost, Ben. Botched circumcision makes man sterile—but $2 million richer. *New York Post*. 2019-11-14, https://nypost.com/2019/11/14/botched-circumcision-makes-man-sterile-but-2-million-richer/.

546 Shteyngart, Gary. A Botched Circumcision and Its Aftermath. *The New Yorker*. 10-11-21, https://www.newyorker.com/magazine/2021/10/11/a-botched-circumcision-and-its-aftermath.

547 Naimer, Sody Sivan Bezalel. Post Circumcision Corona Obliteration. *Journal of Pediatric Urology*. 2020; https://doi.org/10.1016/j.jpurol.2020.04.017.

548 Yevamot 8:2.

549 Stanford Medicine. Complications of Circumcision. 2023, https://med.stanford.edu/newborns/professional-education/circumcision/complications.html.

550 Fleiss, Paul, Hodges, Frederick. *What Your Doctor May Not Tell You About Circumcision*. Hachette Book Group; 2002. p. 2.

551 Petrella, Francis, Ammar, Saloua, El-Sherbiny, Mohamed, Capolicchio, J. P. Total glans amputation after neonatal circumcision. *Urology Case Reports*. 2021/07/01; 37:101624, https://doi.org/10.1016/j.eucr.2021.101624.

552 Akram, Syeda Aiman Akram, Zuber, Ansari, Siddiqa. Delayed gangrene and amputation of penile glans after a religious circumcision in male child—A case report. case-report. *Trop Doct*. 2021-03-09; https://doi.org/10.1177/0049475521998834.

553 Fleiss, Paul, Hodges, Frederick. *What Your Doctor May Not Tell You About Circumcision*. Hachette Book Group; 2002. p. 2.

554 Tawaranurak, N., et al. Successful Pediatric Penile Replantation Following Amputation During Ritual Circumcision: A Case Report and Literature Review. *Am J Case Rep*. Dec 22, 2023; 24:e942448, https://doi.org/10.12659/ajcr.942448.

555 Associated Press. David Reimer, 38, Subject of the John/Joan Case (Published 2004). 2004-05-12, https://www.nytimes.com/2004/05/12/us/david-reimer-38-subject-of-the-john-joan-case.html.

556 Jerusalem Post Staff. Israeli baby requires complex surgery after circumcision gone wrong. *The Jerusalem Post*, https://www.jpost.com/breaking-news/article-716445.

557 Immerman, R. S., Mackey, W. C. A biocultural analysis of circumcision. *Soc Biol*. Fall-Winter 1997; 44(3–4):265–275, https://doi.org/10.1080/19485565.1997.9988953.

558 Wedekind, C., Seebeck, T., Bettens, F., Paepke, A. J. MHC-dependent mate preferences in humans. *Proc Biol Sci*. Jun 22, 1995; 260(1359):245–9, https://doi.org/10.1098/rspb.1995.0087.

559 Everts, Sarah. *The Joy of Sweat: The Strange Science of Perspiration*. 2021. loc. 1239, W. W. Norton and Company.

560 Paraboschi I., Garriboli M. Functions of the Prepuce. *Normal and Abnormal Prepuce*. Springer, Cham; 2020:67, https://doi.org/10.1007/978-3-030-37621-5_7.

561 Guest, Christopher. A Historical and Medical Critique of Circumcision. Accessed March 25, 2016. YouTube, https://www.youtube.com/watch?v=XwZiQyFaAs0&list=PLKuasLinBzLvg-s777BUtAX23LTdDfU6g&index=39&t=0s.

562 Fleiss, Paul, Hodges, Frederick. *What Your Doctor May Not Tell You About Circumcision*. Hachette Book Group; 2002. p. 2.

563 Welk, Blayne, McClure, J. Andrew, Clarke, Collin, Vogt, Kelly, Campbell, Jeffrey. An Opioid Prescription for Men Undergoing Minor Urologic Surgery Is Associated with an Increased Risk of New Persistent Opioid Use. *European Urology*. 2020/01/01; 77(1):68–75, https://doi.org/10.1016/j.eururo.2019.08.031.

564 Newborn Nursery at Lucile Packard Children's Hospital. Complications of Circumcision. Stanford Medicine. 2023, https://med.stanford.edu/newborns/professional-education/circumcision/complications.html.

565 Ritter, Thomas J. *Say No to Circumcision!: 40 Compelling Reasons Why You Should Respect His Birthright and Keep Your Son Whole*. 2020. p. 11–12.

566 Hoffman, Thomas. Male circumcision greatly increases risk of urinary tract problems. *sciencenordiccom*. 2016-12-30; https://www.sciencenordic.com/childrens-health-circumcision-denmark/male-circumcision-greatly-increases-risk-of-urinary-tract-problems/1441376.

567 Margulis, Jennifer. *The Business of Baby*. Scribner, A Division of Simon & Schuster, Inc.; 2013. p. 133.

568 Centers for Disease Control and Prevention. Trends in in-hospital newborn male circumcision—United States, 1999–2010. *MMWR Morbidity and mortality weekly report*. 2011; 60(34):1167–1168.

569 El Bcheraoui, et al. Rates of adverse events associated with male circumcision in U.S. medical settings, 2001 to 2010. *JAMA Pediatr*. 2014; 168(7):625–634, https://doi.org/10.1001/jamapediatrics.2013.5414.

570 Patel, H. The problem of routine circumcision. *Can Med Assoc J*. 1966; 95(11):576–581.

571 Bazmamoun, H., Ghorbanpour, M., Mousavi-Bahar, S. H. Lubrication of circumcision site for prevention of meatal stenosis in children younger than 2 years old. *Urol J*. Fall 2008; 5(4):233–6.

572 Khan, Susankar Kumar Mondal, et al. Use of Lubricant at Meatus and Circumcision Site in Younger Children Prevent Post Circumcision Meatal Stenosis : A Randomized Control Trial. Original Articles. 2013-08-26, https://www.banglajol.info/index.php/JSSMC/article/view/16204.

573 Joudi, Marjan, Fathi, Mehdi, Hiradfar, Mehran. Incidence of asymptomatic meatal stenosis in children following neonatal circumcision. *Journal of Pediatric Urology*. 2011; 7(5):526–528, https://doi.org/10.1016/j.jpurol.2010.08.005.

574 Berry, Carl D., Jr., Cross, Roland R. Urethral Meatal Caliber in Circumcised and Uncircumcised Males. *AMA Journal of Diseases of Children*. 1956; 92(2):152–156, https://doi.org/10.1001/archpedi.1956.02060030146007.

575 Joudi, Marjan, Fathi, Mehdi, Hiradfar, Mehran. Incidence of asymptomatic meatal stenosis in children following neonatal circumcision. *Journal of Pediatric Urology*. 2011; 7(5):526–528, https://doi.org/10.1016/j.jpurol.2010.08.005.

576 Campbell, Meredith. Stenosis of the external urethral meatus. *Journal of Urology*. 1943; 50.

577 Upadhyay, V., Hammodat, H. M., Pease, P. W. Post circumcision meatal stenosis: 12 years' experience. *N Z Med J*. Feb 27 1998; 111(1060):57–8.

578 Mellick, Larry B. Urethral Meatal Stenosis. YouTube, https://www.youtube.com/watch?v=hZLCTx77H3k.

579 Baker, R. L. Newborn Male Circumcision—Needless and dangerous. *Sexual Medicine*. 1979; 3, #11(Nov. 1979):35–36.

580 Schröder, Annette, Farhat, Walid A., Chiasson, David, Wilson, Gregory J., Koyle, Martin A. Serious and Fatal Complications after Neonatal Circumcision. *European Urology Focus*. 2021/12/29; https://doi.org/10.1016/j.euf.2021.12.005.

581 Earp, Brian. Aeonmag. Boys and girls alike; Aeon Essays. 2023; https://aeon.co/essays/are-male-and-female-circumcision-morally-equivalent.

582 Schröder, Annette, Farhat, Walid A., Chiasson, David, Wilson, Gregory J., Koyle, Martin A. Serious and Fatal Complications after Neonatal Circumcision. *European Urology Focus*. 2022/09/01; 8(5):1560–1563, https://doi.org/10.1016/j.euf.2021.12.005.

583 Cunniff, Christopher, Carmack, Janet L., Kirby, Russell S., Fiser, Debra H. Contribution of Heritable Disorders to Mortality in the Pediatric Intensive Care Unit. *Pediatrics*. 1995; 95(5):678–681.

584 Fleiss, Paul, Hodges, Frederick. *What Your Doctor May Not Tell You About Circumcision*. Hachette Book Group; 2002. p. 2.

585 SS, Gellis. Circumcision. *Am J Dis Child*. 1979; 133(10):1079–80.

586 Bollinger, Dan. Lost Boys: An Estimate of U.S. Circumcision-Related Infant Deaths. *Thymos: Journal of Boyhood Studies*. 2010/04/01; 4:78–90.

587 A Scientist Walks into a Bar Podcast. *Preview! The Nutshell Studies and the Mother of Modern Forensics*. A Scientist Walks Into A Bar. June 13, 2020, https://www.youtube.com/watch?v=nw4EKaI4QGU.

588 Ballen, Mr. *It Came From the Basement*. Mr. Ballen Medical Mysteries Podcast. April 23, 2024, https://pca.st/x88997f5.

589 Bollinger, Dan. Lost Boys: An Estimate of U.S. Circumcision-Related Infant Deaths. *Thymos: Journal of Boyhood Studies*. 2010/04/01; 4:78–90.

590 Chapin Georganne, Garrett Echo Montgomery. *The Penis Business: A Memoir*. loc. 3085.

591 Fleiss, Paul, Hodges, Frederick. *What Your Doctor May Not Tell You About Circumcision*. Hachette Book Group; 2002. p. 2.

592 Boston Children's Hospital. Re-circumcision, http://www.childrenshospital.org /conditions-and-treatments/treatments/circumcision/recircumcision.

593 U. S. Department of Health and Human Services. 2020. Penile Curvature (Peyronie's Disease) | NIDDK (2020).

594 Myers, Quinn. What It's Like to Go through Life with A Botched Circumcision. *MelMagazine*, https://melmagazine.com/en-us/story/botched-circumcision -complications-statistics-stories.

595 Gollaher, David. *Circumcision: A History of the World's most Controversial Surgery*. Basic Books, A Member of the Perseus Books Group; 2000. p. 5.

596 Xie, Lin-Hai, Li, Sen-Kai, Li, Qiang. Combined treatment of penile keloid: A troublesome complication after circumcision. *Asian J Androl*. 2013; 15(4):575–576, https:// doi.org/10.1038/aja.2013.23.

597 Fleiss, Paul, Hodges, Frederick. *What Your Doctor May Not Tell You About Circumcision*. Hachette Book Group; 2002. p. 2.

598 Fleiss, Paul, Hodges, Frederick. *What Your Doctor May Not Tell You About Circumcision*. Hachette Book Group; 2002. p. 2.

599 Paraboschi I., Garriboli M. . Functions of the Prepuce. *Normal and Abnormal Prepuce*. Springer, Cham; 2020:67.

600 Boicean, Adrian Haşegan, Ionela, Mihai, Dan, Bratu, et al. Severe Acute Ischemia of Glans Penis after Achieving Treatment with Only Hyperbaric Oxygen Therapy: A Rare Case Report and Systematic Literature Review. Review. *Journal of Personalized Medicine*. 2023-09-12; 13(9):1370, https://doi.org/10.3390/jpm13091370.

601 Justiniano, Ada L. Rivera Cruz, Zasha, F. Vázquez Colón, Hector, Quintero, Cesar Carballo, Cuello, Victor, N. Ortiz. Neonatal Necrotizing Fasciitis after Circumcision: A Case Report and Review of Literature. Review. *Open Journal of Pediatrics*. 2016-03-03; 6(1):29, https://doi.org/doi:10.4236/ojped.2016.61006.

602 Dwyer, Moira, Peffer, Nathan, Fuller, Thomas, Cannon, Glenn. Intraperitoneal Bladder Perforation and Life-threatening Renal Failure in a Neonate Following Circumcision With the Plastibell Device. *Urology*. 2016; 89:134–136, https://doi.org /10.1016/j.urology.2015.11.022.

603 Mor, A., Eshel, G., Aladjem, M., Mundel, G. Tachycardia and heart failure after ritual circumcision. *Arch Dis Child*. 1987; 62(1):80–81, https://doi.org/10.1136/adc.62.1.80.

604 Fleiss, Paul, Hodges, Frederick. *What Your Doctor May Not Tell You About Circumcision*. Hachette Book Group; 2002. p. 2.

605 Bonobo3D. Circumcision—A Mother's Deep Regret. YouTube, https://www.youtube .com/watch?v=uAskbJ7GBok&t=610s.

606 https://www.youtube.com/watch?v=bVBCv5miAO4&list=PLmR7whJ6sRSF47i YcyNvthsXojFaNaayN&index=14.

607 Hospital, Newborn Nursery at Lucile Packard Children's. Complications of Circumcision. Stanford Medicine. 2023, https://med.stanford.edu/newborns/profes- sional-education/circumcision/complications.html.

608 Bigelow, Jim. The Joy of Uncircumcising. 2nd ed. Kearney NE: Morris Publishing; 2002. p. 42.

609 Bonobo3D. Circumcision—A Mother's Deep Regret. Accessed Nov. 25, 2016. YouTube, https://www.youtube.com/watch?v=uAskbJ7GBok&t=610s.

610 Penman, Andrew. *Mirror*. Exposed: the horror statistics behind ritual circumcision of baby boys in the UK. 2023, https://www.mirror.co.uk/news/uk-news/exposed-horrors-ritual-circumcision-baby-28990951.

611 Pascoal, Patricia, et al. The Sexual Pleasure Scale—The Journal of Sexual Medicine. *J Sex Med*. 2017; https://doi.org/doi:10.1016/j.jsxm.2017.04.480.

612 Cold, Cc; J. Taylor. The Prepuce. *Br J Urol*. 1999; 83(1):34–44.

613 Ball, Peter. A Survey of Subjective Foreskin Sensation in 600 Intact Men. In: Denniston G. C. HFM, Milos M. F., ed. *Bodily integrity and the Politics of Circumcision*. 2012, https://link.springer.com/chapter/10.1007/978-1-4020-4916-3_16.

614 Sorrells, M. L., Snyder, J. L., Reiss, M. D., et al. Fine-touch pressure thresholds in the adult penis. *BJU Int*. Apr 2007; 99(4):864–9, https://doi.org/10.1111/j.1464-410X.2006.06685.x.

615 Fleiss, Paul, Hodges, Frederick. *What Your Doctor May Not Tell You About Circumcision*. Hachette Book Group; 2002. p. 2.

616 Fink, Kenneth S., Carson, Culley C., DeVellis, Robert F. Adult circumcision outcomes study: effect on erectile function, penile sensitivity, sexual activity and satisfaction. *J Urol*. 2002; 167(5):2113–2116.

617 Sorrells, M. L., Snyder, J. L., Reiss, M. D., et al. Fine-touch pressure thresholds in the adult penis. *BJU Int*. Apr 2007; 99(4):864–9, https://doi.org/10.1111/j.1464-410X.2006.06685.x.

618 Yang, D. M., Lin, H., Zhang, B., Guo, W. Circumcision affects glans penis vibration perception threshold. *Zhonghua Nan Ke Xue*. Apr 2008; 14(4):328–30, https://pubmed.ncbi.nlm.nih.gov/18481425/.

619 Foley, John M., M.D. The unkindest cut of all. *FACT magazine*. 3:4, July–Aug, 1966. p. 2–9.

620 Bronselaer, Guy A., Schober, Justine M., Meyer-Bahlburg, Heino F. L., T'Sjoen, Guy, Vlietinck, Robert, Hoebeke, Piet B. Male circumcision decreases penile sensitivity as measured in a large cohort. *BJU Int*. 2013; 111(5):820–827, https://doi.org/10.1111/j.1464-410X.2012.11761.x.

621 Boyle, G. J., Bensley, G. A. Adverse sexual and psychological effects of male infant circumcision. *Psychol Rep*. 2001; 88(3 Pt 2):1105–1106, https://doi.org/10.2466/pro.2001.88.3c.1105.

622 Sorrells, M. L., Snyder, J. L., Reiss, M. D., et al. Fine-touch pressure thresholds in the adult penis. *BJU Int*. Apr 2007; 99(4):864–9, https://doi.org/10.1111/j.1464-410X.2006.06685.x.

623 Frisch, Morten, Lindholm, Morten, Grønbæk, Morten. Male circumcision and sexual function in men and women: A survey-based, cross-sectional study in Denmark. *Int J Epidemiol*. 2011; 40(5):1367–1381, https://doi.org/10.1093/ije/dyr104.

624 Rowland, D., McMahon, C. G., Abdo, C., et al. Disorders of orgasm and ejaculation in men. *J Sex Med*. Apr 2010; 7(4 Pt 2):1668–86, https://doi.org/10.1111/j.1743-6109.2010.01782.x.

625 Sorrells, M. L., Snyder, J. L., Reiss, M. D., et al. Fine-touch pressure thresholds in the adult penis. *BJU Int*. Apr 2007; 99(4):864–9, https://doi.org/10.1111/j.1464-410X.2006.06685.x.

626 Senkul, T., Işer, I. C., şen, B., KarademIr, K., Saraçoğlu, F., Erden, D. Circumcision in adults: effect on sexual function. *Urology*. Jan 2004; 63(1):155–8, https://doi.org/10.1016/j.urology.2003.08.035.

627 Senol, M. G., Sen, B., Karademir, K., Sen, H., Saraçoğlu, M. The effect of male circumcision on pudendal evoked potentials and sexual satisfaction. *Acta Neurol Belg*. Sep 2008; 108(3):90–93.

628 Taves, Donald R. The intromission function of the foreskin. *Medical Hypotheses*. 2020; 59(2).

629 Shen, Zhoujun, Chen, Shanwen, Zhu, Chunxia, Wan, Qun, Chen, Zhaodian. Erectile function evaluation after adult circumcision. *Zhonghua Nan Ke Xue*. 2004; 10(1):18–19.

630 Fink, Kenneth S., Carson, Culley C., DeVellis, Robert F. Adult circumcision outcomes study: effect on erectile function, penile sensitivity, sexual activity and satisfaction. *J Urol*. 2002; 167(5):2113–2116.

631 Bronselaer, Guy A., Schober, Justine M., Meyer-Bahlburg, Heino F. L., T'Sjoen, Guy, Vlietinck, Robert, Hoebeke, Piet B. Male circumcision decreases penile sensitivity as measured in a large cohort. *BJU Int*. 2013; 111(5):820–827, https://doi.org/10.1111/j.1464-410X.2012.11761.x.

632 Solinis I, Yiannaki A. Does circumcision improve couple's sex life? *Journal of Mens Health and Gender*. 2007; 4(3):361.

633 Bossio, J. A., Pukall, C. F., Steele, S. A review of the current state of the male circumcision literature. *J Sex Med*. Dec 2014; 11(12):2847–64, https://doi.org/10.1111/jsm.12703.

634 Bossio, Jennifer A. *Examining Sexual Correlates of Neonatal Circumcision*. Queen's University; 2015, https://qspace.library.queensu.ca/items/43b2e9b3-f73e-4967-a2c7-5e4e8a1dd738.

635 O'Hara, Jeffrey, O'Hara, Kristen. *Sex As Nature Intended It: The Most Important Thing You Need to Know About Making Love, But No One Could Tell You Until Now*. 2nd ed. Turning Point Publications. loc. 942. Hereafter cited as O'Hara.

636 Fink, Kenneth S., Carson, Culley C., and DeVellis, Robert F. Adult circumcision outcomes study: effect on erectile function, penile sensitivity, sexual activity and satisfaction. *J Urol*. 2002; 167(5):2113–2116.

637 Shen, Zhoujun, Chen, Shanwen, Zhu, Chunxia, Wan, Qun, Chen, Zhaodian. Erectile function evaluation after adult circumcision. *Zhonghua Nan Ke Xue*. 2004; 10(1):18–19.

638 Bollinger, Dan, Van Howe, Robert. Alexithymia and Circumcision Trauma: A Preliminary Investigation. *International Journal of Men's Health*. 2011/05/01; 10:184–195.

639 Tang, W. S., Khoo, E. M. Prevalence and correlates of premature ejaculation in a primary care setting: A preliminary cross-sectional study. *J Sex Med*. Jul 2011; 8(7):2071–78, https://doi.org/10.1111/j.1743-6109.2011.02280.x.

640 Elizabeth, Selvin, Burnett, Arthur, Platz, Elizabeth. Prevalence and Risk Factors for Erectile Dysfunction in the US. *The American Journal of Medicine*. 2007/02/01; 120(2):151–157, https://doi.org/10.1016/j.amjmed.2006.06.010.

641 Shen, Zhoujun, Chen, Shanwen, Zhu, Chunxia, Wan, Qun, Chen, Zhaodian. Erectile function evaluation after adult circumcision. *Zhonghua Nan Ke Xue*. 2004; 10(1):18–19.

642 Lang, David. Implicit Catholic Teaching against Non-Therapeutic Child Circumcision—Catholics Against Circumcision. Updated 2021-08-10, https://www .catholicsagainstcircumcision.org/implicit-catholic-teaching-against-non-therapeutic -child-circumcision/.

643 Tang, W. S., Khoo, E. M. Prevalence and correlates of premature ejaculation in a primary care setting: A preliminary cross-sectional study. *J Sex Med*. Jul 2011; 8(7):2071–78, https://doi.org/10.1111/j.1743-6109.2011.02280.x.

644 Masood, S., Patel, H. R. H., Himpson, R. C., Palmer, J. H., Mufti, G. R., Sheriff, M. K. M. Penile sensitivity and sexual satisfaction after circumcision: Are we informing men correctly? *Urol Int*. 2005; 75(1):62–66, https://doi.org/10.1159/000085930.

645 Roach, Mary. *Bonk: The Curious Coupling of Science and Sex*. Reprint edition (April 6, 2009), W. W. Norton & Company; p. 41, https://www.amazon.com/dp/B003 M5IGE2.

646 Anderson, Wendy Love. *The Goy of Sex*. New York, NY: NYU Press; 2009.

647 Tahtali, Ibrahim Nuvit. The Relationship between age of circumcision and premature ejaculation. 2021, https://openurl.ebsco.com/EPDB%3Agcd%3A7%3A20507959 /detailv2?sid=ebsco%3Aplink%3Ascholar&id=ebsco%3Agcd%3A152087272&crl=c.

648 O'Hara, loc. 942.

649 Taylor, J. R., Lockwood, A. P., Taylor, A. J. The prepuce: specialized mucosa of the penis and its loss to circumcision. *Br J Urol*. 1996; 77(2):291–295, https://doi.org /10.1046/j.1464-410x.1996.85023.x.

650 Podnar, S. RE: Clinical elicitation of the penilo-cavernosus reflex in circumcised men. *BJU Int*. Sep 2012; 110(5):E161, https://doi.org/10.1111/j.1464-410X.2012.11250_2.x.

651 Bigelow, Jim. Uncircumcising: undoing the effects of an ancient practice in a modern world. *Mothering*. 1994 (Summer):56–61, https://www.cirp.org/library/restoration /bigelow1/.

652 S., Pertot. Sensitivity is the rising issue. *Australian Doctor*,. 1994.;(25 November).

653 https://foreskinrestoration.men/.

654 Israel Story Podcast. *Lost and Found—Part II*, https://www.israelstory.org/episode /lost-and-found-part-ii/. November 15, 2021.

655 Gupta, R., Mehta, S., Gupta, R. A Novel Procedure of Prepuce Reconstruction Customized to the Religious Needs of Some Individuals. *Indian J Plast Surg*. Apr 2021; 54(2):114–117, https://doi.org/10.1055/s-0041-1731621.

656 Song, B., Hou, Z. H., Liu, Q. L., Qian, W. P. [Penile frenulum lengthening for premature ejaculation]. *Zhonghua Nan Ke Xue*. Feb 2015; 21(2):149–52.

657 Gupta, R., Mehta, S., Gupta, R. A Novel Procedure of Prepuce Reconstruction Customized to the Religious Needs of Some Individuals. *Indian J Plast Surg*. Apr 2021; 54(2):114–117, https://doi.org/10.1055/s-0041-1731621.

658 https://www.foregen.org/.

659 Kim, Daisik, Pang, Myung-Geol. The effect of male circumcision on sexuality. *BJU Int*. 2007; 99(3):619–622, https://doi.org/10.1111/j.1464-410X.2006.06646.x.

660 Kim, Myung-Geol PangSae Chul KimDaiSik. Male Circumcision in South Korea | SpringerLink. In: Denniston GHFMM, ed. *Understanding Circumcision*. SpringerLink; 2020.

661 Denniston Gc, Hill G. Circumcision in adults: effect on sexual function. *Urology.* 2004; 64(6):1267.

662 https://www.haaretz.com/israel-news/.premium.MAGAZINE-they-felt -pressured-to-get-circumcised-after-moving-to-israel-they-now-regret-it-1.8227063.

663 Bronselaer, Guy A., Schober, Justine M., Meyer-Bahlburg, Heino F. L., T'Sjoen, Guy, Vlietinck, Robert, Hoebeke, Piet B. Male circumcision decreases penile sensitivity as measured in a large cohort. *BJU Int.* 2013; 111(5):820–827, https://doi.org/10.1111 /j.1464-410X.2012.11761.x.

664 Zwang, G. *Sexual Mutilations: A Human Tragedy.* 1997. Loc. 2173, https://www .amazon.com/Sexual-Mutilations-Tragedy-Defense-Research-ebook/dp/B000SEP E8Q/ref=sr_1_9?dchild=1&keywords=marilyn+milos&qid=1598373261&sr=8-9.

665 Zilbergeld, Bernie, PhD. *Male Sexuality: A guide to sexual fulfillment.* Boston: Little, Brown and Co.; 1978. p. 3–4.

666 Fugl-Meyer, K. S., Oberg, K., Lundberg, P. O., Lewin, B., Fugl-Meyer, A. On orgasm, sexual techniques, and erotic perceptions in 18- to 74-year-old Swedish women. *J Sex Med.* Jan 2006; 3(1):56–68, https://doi.org/10.1111/j.1743-6109.2005.00170.x.

667 Haavio-Mannila, E., Kontula, O. Correlates of increased sexual satisfaction. *Arch Sex Behav.* Aug 1997; 26(4):399–419, https://doi.org/10.1023/a:1024591318836.

668 Haning, R. V., O'Keefe, S. L., Randall, E. J., Kommor, M. J., Baker, E., Wilson, R. Intimacy, orgasm likelihood, and conflict predict sexual satisfaction in heterosexual male and female respondents. *J Sex Marital Ther.* Mar-Apr 2007; 33(2):93–113, https://doi.org/10.1080/00926230601098449.

669 Philippsohn, S., Hartmann, U. Determinants of sexual satisfaction in a sample of German women. *J Sex Med.* Apr 2009; 6(4):1001–1010, https://doi.org/10.1111/j.1743 -6109.2008.00989.x.

670 Santtila, P., Wager, I., Witting, K., et al. Discrepancies between sexual desire and sexual activity: gender differences and associations with relationship satisfaction. *J Sex Marital Ther.* 2008; 34(1):31–44, https://doi.org/10.1080/00926230701620548.

671 Davey Smith, G., Frankel, S., Yarnell, J. Sex and death: Are they related? Findings from the Caerphilly Cohort Study. *BMJ.* Dec 20–27 1997; 315(7123):1641–4, https://doi .org/10.1136/bmj.315.7123.1641.

672 Sm, G., Gallup G., Burch, R. L., Platek. Does semen have antidepressant properties? *Archives of sexual behavior.* 2002 Jun 2002; 31(3), https://doi.org/10.1023/a:101525 7004839.

673 Roach, Mary. *Bonk: The Curious Coupling of Science and Sex.* Reprint edition (April 6, 2009), W. W. Norton & Company; 2009. p. 41, https://www.amazon.com/dp /B003M5IGE2.

674 Killen, Amy. *How to Improve Your Sexual Pleasure.* Broken Brain Podcast. July 13, 2020.

675 Rider, Jennifer R., Wilson, Kathryn M., Sinnott, Jennifer A., et al., Ejaculation Frequency and Risk of Prostate Cancer: Updated Results with an Additional Decade of Follow-up. *European Urology.* 2016/12/01; 70(6):974–982, https://doi.org/10.1016 /j.eururo.2016.03.027.

676 Charnetski, C. J., Brennan, F. X. Sexual frequency and salivary immunoglobulin A (IgA). *Psychol Rep.* Jun 2004; 94(3 Pt 1):839–44, https://doi.org/10.2466/pr0.94.3 .839-844.

677 Malik, Rena. Sciences proves that ejaculating more often reduces your risk of CANCER?! A Urologist explains, https://www.youtube.com/watch?v=ZYhZMsvBWSU.

678 Klotz, Charles. 1,153 Fun Facts: To Leave You Astounded. 2021. loc. 663.

679 yourwholebaby.org. The Blog @ Your Whole Baby,, https://www.yourwholebaby.org/blog/without-his-foreskin.

680 Ahituv, Netta. Even in Israel, More and More Parents Choose Not to Circumcise Their Sons. *Haaretz*. June 14, 2012, https://www.haaretz.com/even-in-israel-more-and-more-parents-choose-not-to-circumcise-1.5178506.

681 https://www.haaretz.com/israel-news/.premium.MAGAZINE-they-felt-pressured-to-get-circumcised-after-moving-to-israel-they-now-regret-it-1.8227063.

682 Bigelow, Jim. The Joy of Uncircumcising! 2nd ed. Kearney NE: Morris Publishing; 2002. p. 15.

683 Ritter, Thomas J. *Say No to Circumcision!: 40 Compelling Reasons Why You Should Respect His Birthright and Keep Your Son Whole*. 2020. p. 11–12.

684 O'Hara, loc. 942.

685 O'Hara, loc. 942.

686 O'Hara, loc. 942.

687 Morris, Brian, Krieger, John. Does Male Circumcision Affect Sexual Function, Sensitivity, or Satisfaction?—A Systematic Review. *J Sex Med*. 2013/08/12; 10, https://doi.org/10.1111/jsm.12293.

688 Baskin, Laurence. Neonatal circumcision: Risks and benefits. *UpToDate*. Jan 2024.

689 Roach, Mary. *Bonk: The Curious Coupling of Science and Sex*. Reprint edition (April 6, 2009), W. W. Norton & Company; 2009. p. 41, https://www.amazon.com/dp/B003M5IGE2.

690 Bartley, Katie, Bossio, Jennifer A., Pukall, Caroline F. You either have it or you don't: The impact of male circumcision status on sexual partners. *The Canadian Journal of Human Sexuality*. 2015; 24(2):104–119, https://psycnet.apa.org/record/2015-45299-004.

691 Mao, L., Templeton, D. J., Crawford, J., et al. Does circumcision make a difference to the sexual experience of gay men? Findings from the Health in Men (HIM) cohort. *J Sex Med*. Nov 2008; 5(11):2557–61, https://doi.org/10.1111/j.1743-6109.2008.00845.x.

692 Martin, Robert D. Masturbation: Self-Abuse or Biological Necessity? 2007, https://www.psychologytoday.com/blog/how-we-do-it/201711/masturbation-self-abuse-or-biological-necessity.

693 Habash, Gabe. Why Is the Penis Shaped Like That? PW Talks with Jesse Bering. *Publisher's Weekly*. article no longer available online.

694 Kim, Daisik, Pang, Myung-Geol. The effect of male circumcision on sexuality. *BJU Int*. 2007; 99(3):619–622, https://doi.org/10.1111/j.1464-410X.2006.06646.x.

695 Bensley, G. A., Boyle, G. J. Physical, Sexual, and Psychological Effects of Male Infant Circumcision: A New Preputial Structure. In: Denniston GHFMM, ed. *Understanding Circumcision*. SpringerLink; 2020:218.

696 Fleiss, Paul, Hodges, Frederick. *What Your Doctor May Not Tell You About Circumcision*. Hachette Book Group; 2002. p. 2.

697 AsapSCIENCE. Is Masturbation Good For You? YouTube, https://www.youtube.com/watch?v=GU3JqoUDkjA.

698 UroChannel. The healthy penis' ultimate maintenance program. YouTube, https://www.youtube.com/watch?v=8lI__-HBX-I&list=PLKuasLinBzLvg-s777BUtAX23L TdDfU6g&index=88&t=120s.

699 Park, Jong Kwan, Doo, A. Ram, Kim, Joo Heung, et al. Prospective investigation of penile length with newborn male circumcision and second to fourth digit ratio. *Can Urol Assoc J.* Sep-Oct 2016; 10(9–10):E296-E299, https://doi.org/10.5489/cuaj.3590.

700 Ritter, Thomas J. *Say No to Circumcision!: 40 Compelling Reasons Why You Should Respect His Birthright and Keep Your Son Whole.* 2020. p. 11–12.

701 Bronselaer, Guy A., et al. Male circumcision decreases penile sensitivity as measured in a large cohort. *BJU Int.* 2013; 111(5):820–827, https://doi.org/10.1111/j.1464-410X .2012.11761.x.

702 Zwang, G. *Sexual Mutilations: A Human Tragedy.* 1997. Loc. 2173, https://www .amazon.com/Sexual-Mutilations-Tragedy-Defense-Research-ebook/dp/B000SEPE8 Q/ref=sr_1_9?dchild=1&keywords=marilyn+milos&qid=1598373261&sr=8-9.

703 Frisch, Morten, Simonsen, Jacob. Ritual circumcision and risk of autism spectrum disorder in 0- to 9-year-old boys: national cohort study in Denmark. *J R Soc Med.* 2015; 108(7):266–279, https://doi.org/10.1177/0141076814565942.

704 John, Timothy. Facing Circumcision: Eight Physicians Tell Their Stories. 1998. YouTube, https://www.youtube.com/watch?v=z_ExlVUGsig.

705 Carmack, Adrienne. X post, https://x.com/intactamerica/status/1509454205135765507 /photo/1.

706 Bonobo3D. Doctor Denounces Circumcision of Children. YouTube, https://www .youtube.com/watch?v=xgGeOvSgPu4.

707 Matar, Lea, Zhu, Julia, Chen, Robert T., Gust, Deborah A. Medical risks and benefits of newborn male circumcision in the United States: physician perspectives. *J Int Assoc Provid AIDS Care.* Jan-Feb 2015; 14(1):33–39, https://doi.org/10.1177/2325957414 535975.

708 Milos, M. F., Kirkwood, Judy. *Please Don't Cut the Baby: A Nurse's Memoir.* loc. 784.

709 Deacon, Matthew, Muir, Gordon. What is the medical evidence on non-therapeutic child circumcision? *International Journal of Impotence Research.* 2022/01/08; https://doi.org/10.1038/s41443-021-00502-y.

710 Australian Institute of Health and Welfare. *A picture of Australia's children 2009.* 2009, https://www.aihw.gov.au/reports/children-youth/picture-australias-children-2009.

711 *Kenneth Lipman's website list of circumcision pros and cons*, https://kennethlipman .com/circumcision-pros-vs-cons/.

712 Frisch, Morten, Lindholm, Morten, Grønbæk, Morten. Male circumcision and sexual function in men and women: A survey-based, cross-sectional study in Denmark. *Int J Epidemiol.* 2011; 40(5):1367–1381, https://doi.org/10.1093/ije/dyr104.

713 O'Hara, loc. 942.

714 Delamothe, Tony. Round the bend. *BMJ.* 2019; 367:l6654, https://doi.org/10.1136 /bmj.l6654.

715 O'Hara, loc. 930.

716 O'Hara, loc. 930.

717 O'Hara, loc. 2268.

718 O'Hara, loc. 796.

719 O'Hara, loc. 4604.

720 O'Hara, loc. 1954.

721 O'Hara, loc. 1952.

722 O'Hara, loc. 1956.

723 Cleveland Clinic. Delayed Ejaculation Disorder: Causes & Treatment, https://my .clevelandclinic.org/health/diseases/22125-delayed-ejaculation.

724 O'Hara, loc. 2308.

725 O'Hara, loc. 1513.

726 O'Hara, loc. 2325.

727 Bigelow, Jim. The Joy of Uncircumcizing. 2nd ed. Kearney NE: Morris Publishing; 2002. p. 10.

728 Bigelow, Jim. The Joy of Uncircumcizing. 2nd ed. Kearney NE: Morris Publishing; 2002. p. 10.

729 Pollack, Miriam. Circumcision: Identity, Gender, and Power. *Tikkun*, https://www .tikkun.org/circumcision-identity-gender-and-power.

730 O'Hara, K., O'Hara, J. The effect of male circumcision on the sexual enjoyment of the female partner. *BJU Int*. Jan 1999; 83 Suppl 1:79–84, https://doi.org/10.1046/j.1464 -410x.1999.0830s1079.x.

731 Cortés-González, Jeff R., Arratia-Maqueo, Jorge A., Gómez-Guerra, Lauro S. Does circumcision has an effect on female's perception of sexual satisfaction? *Rev Invest Clin*. May-Jun 2008; 60(3):227–230.

732 Goldman, Ronald. *Circumcision, The Hidden Trauma : How an American Cultural Practice Affects Infants and Ultimately Us All*. Vanguard; 1997. p. 110.

733 Ritter, Thomas J. *Say No to Circumcision!: 40 Compelling Reasons Why You Should Respect His Birthright and Keep Your Son Whole*. 2020. p. 15-2.

734 Erickson, John A. Does Male Circumcision Help Spread AIDS? http://www.sexually mutilatedchild.org/does-c.htm.

735 Goodman, J. Jewish circumcision: An alternative perspective. *Br J Urol*. 1999; 83(1):22–27.

736 Pollack, Miriam. *Sexual Mutilations: A Human Tragedy*. 1997. Loc. 3958, https:// www.amazon.com/Sexual-Mutilations-Tragedy-Defense-Research-ebook/dp /B000SEPE8Q/ref=sr_1_9?dchild=1&keywords=marilyn+milos&qid=159837326 1&sr=8-9.

737 Keats, Jonathan. 20 Things You Didn't Know About Learning. *Discover*. September/ October 2020, https://www.discovermagazine.com/mind/20-things-you-didnt-know -about-learning.

738 Marshall, Richard E., Stratton, William C., Moore, Jo Ann, Boxerman, Stuart B. Circumcision I: Effects upon newborn behavior. *Infant Behavior and Development*. 1980/01/01; 3:1–14, https://doi.org/10.1016/S0163-6383(80)80003-8.

739 Van Howe, Robert S. A Cost-Utility Analysis of Neonatal Circumcision. *Medical Decision Making*. 2004/11/01; 24(6):584–601, https://doi.org/10.1177/02729 89X04271039.

740 Chapin Georganne, Garrett Echo Montgomery. *The Penis Business: A Memoir*. loc. 3085.

741 Van Howe, Robert S. A Cost-Utility Analysis of Neonatal Circumcision. *Medical Decision Making*. 2004/11/01; 24(6):584–601, https://doi.org/10.1177/0272989X0 4271039.

742 Pieretti-Vanmarcke, Rafael V. Pieretti, Allan, M. Goldstein, Rafael. Late complications of newborn circumcision: A common and avoidable problem. *Pediatric Surgery International*. 2010-02-14; 26(5):515–518, https://doi.org/doi:10.1007/s00383-010 -2566-9.

743 Margulis, Jennifer. *The Business of Baby*. Scribner, A Division of Simon & Schuster, Inc.; 2013. p. 133.

744 MDSave. National Average, https://www.mdsave.com/f/procedure/pediatric -circumcision/94705?q=Pediatric+Circumcision&name=Pediatric%20 Circumcision&latLng=37.86106,-122.25649&city=Berkeley&state=California& zip=94705.

745 Bobrow, Emily. The industrialized world is turning against circumcision. It's time for the US to consider doing the same. *Quartz*. Jan. 17, 2017, https://qz.com/885018/why -is-circumcision-so-popular-in-the-us/.

746 U.S. Bureau of Labor Statistics. CPI Inflation Calculator, https://www.bls.gov/data /inflation_calculator.htm.

747 Haaretz. Dec. 7, 2019. They Felt Pressured to Get Circumcised After Moving to Israel. They Now Regret It, https://www.haaretz.com/israel-news/.premium.MAGAZINE -they-felt-pressured-to-get-circumcised-after-moving-to-israel-they-now-regret-it -1.8227063.

748 Personal communication with Dr. James Snyder regarding another physician.

749 Bollinger, Dan. Lost Boys: An Estimate of U.S. Circumcision-Related Infant Deaths. *Thymos: Journal of Boyhood Studies*. 2010/04/01; 4:78–90.

750 Margulis, Jennifer. *The Business of Baby*. Scribner, A Division of Simon & Schuster, Inc.; 2013. p. 133.

751 Bollinger, Dan. The Penis-Care Information Gap: Preventing Improper Care of Intact Boys. *Thymos: Journal of Boyhood Studies*. 2007/07/01; 1:205–219, https://doi.org /10.3149/thy.0205.219.

752 Zambrano Navia, Mateo, Jacobson, Deborah L., Balmert, Lauren C., et al. State-Level Public Insurance Coverage and Neonatal Circumcision Rates. *Pediatrics*. 2020/11/; 146(5) https://doi.org/10.1542/peds.2020-1475.

753 Leibowitz, A. A., Desmond, K., Belin, T. Determinants and policy implications of male circumcision in the United States. *Am J Public Health*. Jan 2009; 99(1):138–45, https://doi.org/10.2105/ajph.2008.134403.

754 Linfield, Rebecca Y., Wendling, Ryan, Slusky, David J. G. The 1982 Medicaid Funding Cessation for Circumcision in California and Circumcision Rates. *AIDS and Behavior*. 2022-11-07:1–6, https://doi.org/doi:10.1007/s10461-022-03896-y.

755 Child Circumcision: An Elephant in the Hospital. YouTube, https://www.youtube .com/watch?v=Ceht-3xu84I.

756 C., Remi. Here's where foreskins are sold. Yelp.com, https://www.yelp.com/topic/san -francisco-heres-where-foreskins-are-sold.

757 Losquadro, Anthony. Circumcision in America: Are baby boys' foreskins for sale? *"mediumcom."* 2021-02-21, https://anthonylosquadro.medium.com/circumcision -in-america-are-baby-boys-foreskins-for-sale-e0b79fadc8cb.

758 ScienceNews. Scientists grew living human skin around a robotic finger. 2022-06-09; https://www.sciencenews.org/article/robotic-finger-human-skin-self-healing.

759 Oliveira, Thomaz, Costa, Ilana, Marinho, Victor, et al. Human foreskin fibroblasts: from waste bag to important biomedical applications. *Journal of Clinical Urology.* 2018; 11(6):385–394, https://doi.org/10.1177/2051415818761526.

760 Saarman, Emily. How We Got the Controversial HPV Vaccine. *Discover Magazine.* May 16, 2007, https://www.discovermagazine.com/health/how-we-got-the -controversial-hpv-vaccine.

761 Margulis, Jennifer. *The Business of Baby.* Scribner, A Division of Simon & Schuster, Inc.; 2013. p. 133.

762 C., Remi. Here's where foreskins are sold. Yelp.com, https://www.yelp.com/topic /san-francisco-heres-where-foreskins-are-sold.

763 Margulis, Jennifer. *The Business of Baby.* Scribner, A Division of Simon & Schuster, Inc.; 2013. p. 133.

764 C., Remi. Here's where foreskins are sold. Yelp.com, https://www.yelp.com/topic /san-francisco-heres-where-foreskins-are-sold.

765 Aldag, Caroline, Nogueira Teixeira, Diana, Leventhal, Phillip S. Skin rejuvenation using cosmetic products containing growth factors, cytokines, and matrikines: A review of the literature. *Clin Cosmet Investig Dermatol.* 2016; 9:411–419, https://doi .org/10.2147/CCID.S116158.

766 Barrie, Josh. Foreskin facials: The truth behind the penis-based beauty regime. *inewscouk*, https://inews.co.uk/inews-lifestyle/people/foreskin-facial-kate-beckinsale -penis-skin-treatment-201331.

767 Malamut, Melissa. The 'Baby Foreskin Facial' Is a Real Thing. *Boston Magazine,* https://www.bostonmagazine.com/health/2015/04/14/baby-foreskin-facial-boston -hydrafacial/.

768 Margulis, Jennifer. *The Business of Baby.* Scribner, A Division of Simon & Schuster, Inc.; 2013. p. 133.

769 Makary, Marty. *The Price We Pay: What Broke American Health Care—and How to Fix It.* Bloomsbury Publishing; 2019. loc. 3320, https://www.amazon.com/dp /B07MXPJ33B.

770 Losquadro, Anthony. Circumcision in America: Are baby boys' foreskins for sale? *"mediumcom."* 2021-02-21, https://anthonylosquadro.medium.com/circumcision -in-america-are-baby-boys-foreskins-for-sale-e0b79fadc8cb.

771 Bollinger, Dan. *High Cost of Circumcision $5.7 Billion Annually.* 2022.

772 A Groundbreaking Intact America Survey. 2020-11-16, 2020, https://intactamerica .org/press-release-having-a-baby-boy-get-ready-for-the-circumcision-sellers/.

773 Bonobo3D. Circumcision—A Mother's Deep Regret. YouTube, https://www.youtube .com/watch?v=uAskbJ7GB0k.

774 Brown, Maressa. Mom Gets 'Circumcision-Shamed' at Her OB-GYN & Honestly, She's Pissed. Cafemom blog, https://thestir.cafemom.com/pregnancy/225357/mom -faces-circumcision-shaming-nurse.

775 Zeimet, Sarah. Voices—Sarah Zeimet—Intact America. 2021. Blog, https://intact america.org/voices-sarah-zeimet/.

776 Milos, M. F., Kirkwood, Judy. *Please Don't Cut the Baby: A Nurse's Memoir*. loc. 784. Lucid House Publishing LLC.

777 Nunn, Gary. Foreskin reclaimers: the 'intactivists' fighting infant male circumcision. *The Guardian*. July 20, 2019.

778 Losquadro, Anthony. Dr. Health Radio Fast Moving Discussion on Circumcision. The Circumcision Chronicles Uncut Podcast 2019.

779 Hill, George. Protection of Infant Boys from Wrongful Circumcision in American Hospitals, http://www.cirp.org/pages/parents/protection/.

780 Los Angeles County Superior Court No. SOC 36797. Verdict Report 24. 1979.

781 Llewellyn, David J. Legal remedies for penile torts. *The Complete Mother*. 1995; 40(16.)

782 Reinert, Sue. $80,000 settlement to circumcised boy. *The Patriot Ledger*. January 5, 2001.

783 Meddings, Jonathan. *The Final Cut: The truth about circumcision*. 2022. p. 105, https:// www.amazon.com/Final-Cut-truth-about-circumcision/dp/0645368202/ref=sr_1_ 1?crid=1I3QHK0OIRK4M&keywords=the+final+cut+circumcision&qid=1702883 041&s=books&sprefix=the+final+cut+circumcision%2Cstripbooks%2C121&sr=1-1.

784 Drash, Michael. Circumcising human subjects: An evaluation of experimental foreskin amputation using the Declaration of Helsinki. *Bioethics*. 2019; 33(3):383–388, https://doi.org/10.1111/bioe.12566.

785 Attorneys for the Rights of the Child. Human Rights Violations Table, https://www .arclaw.org/resources/human-rights-violations-table.

786 American Academy of Pediatrics Task Force on Circumcision. Informed Consent, Parental Permission, and Assent in Pediatric Practice. *Pediatrics*. 1995; 95(2):314–317.

787 The Brussels Collaboration on Body Integrity. Medically Unnecessary Genital Cutting and the Rights of the Child: Moving Toward Consensus. *The American Journal of Bioethics*. 2019/10/03; 19(10):17–28, https://doi.org/10.1080/15265161.201 9.1643945.

788 Earp, B. D. Male or female genital cutting: why 'health benefits' are morally irrelevant. *J Med Ethics*. Jan 18, 2021; https://doi.org/10.1136/medethics-2020-106782.

789 Washington, Harriet A. *Carte Blanche: The Erosion of Medical Consent—Kindle edition by Washington, Harriet A. Professional & Technical Kindle eBooks @ Amazon.com.* 2021. loc. 88, https://amazon.com/Carte-Blanche-Erosion-Medical-Consent -ebook/dp/B08MCC43CK/ref=sr_1_1?dchild=1&keywords=carte+blanche +harriet+washington&qid=1625930236&sr=8-1.

790 Personal communication.

791 Svoboda, J. Steven. Circumcision of male infants as a human rights violation. *J Med Ethics*. 2013; 39(7):469–474, https://doi.org/10.1136/medethics-2012-101229.

792 California Court of Appeal. Tortorella v. Castro. No B184043. Second District, Division 32006.

793 Attorneys for the Rights of the Child blog. Taxpayers Sue Massachusetts Medicaid. July 22, 2020, https://www.arclaw.org/news/taxpayers-sue-massachusetts-medicaid.

794 Adler, Peter W. Is it lawful to use Medicaid to pay for circumcision? *J Law Med*. 2011; 19(2):335–353.

795 Massachusetts G.L. c. 29, § 63.

796 Attorneys for the Rights of the Child. LAVINE VS AAP, https://www.circumcision isafraud.com/docket-mer-l-000272-21.

797 Timmins, Annemarie. Bill ending Medicaid coverage for elective circumcisions fails. New Hampshire Bulletin, https://newhampshirebulletin.com/briefs/bill-ending -medicaid-coverage-for-elective-circumcisions-fails/.

798 Peter W. Adler, Robert Van Howe Travis Wisdom Felix Daase. *Is Circumcision a Fraud?* 2021, https://ww3.lawschool.cornell.edu/research/JLPP/upload/Adler-et -al-final.pdf.

799 Earp, Brian. Why Was the U.S. Ban on Female Genital Mutilation Ruled Unconstitutional, and What Does This Have to Do With Male Circumcision? *Ethics Medicine and Public Health*. 2020/07/01; https://doi.org/10.1016/j.jemep.2020.100533.

800 Reporter, Malawi. Children in Malawi demand compensation over circumcision Malawi 24 | Latest News from Malawi. *Malawi24*. 2023-11-18, https://malawi24. com/2023/11/18/children-in-malawi-demand-compensation-over-circumcision/.

801 news@thelocal.dk. Danish doctors come out against circumcision. *The Local*. 2016-12-05, https://www.thelocal.dk/20161205/danish-doctors-come-out-against -circumcision.

802 KNMG. *The non-therapeutic circumcision of male minors*. 2010. May 27, 2010, https:// www.knmg.nl/download/non-therapeutic-circumcision-of-male-minors-knmg -viewpoint.

803 Scott, Kellie. Should we circumcise our son just because his dad is? *ABC Everyday*. 2021-03-22, https://www.abc.net.au/everyday/should-we-circumcise-our-son-just -because-his-dad-is/10001221.

804 intaction.org. Blog. German Pediatric Association condemns infant circumcision. @intaction1. Updated 2012-12-29, https://intaction.org/german-pediatric-association -condemns-infant-circumcision-2/.

805 British Medical Association. *Non-therapeutic male circumcision (NTMC) of children— practical guidance for doctors*. 2019, https://www.bma.org.uk/media/1847/bma -non-therapeutic-male-circumcision-of-children-guidance-2019.pdf.

806 Canadian Medical Assocation. Neonatal circumcision revisited. Fetus and Newborn Committee, Canadian Paediatric Society. *CMAJ*. 1996; 154(6):769–780.

807 Dua, Sumeet. KevinMD.com. Blog. Why male circumcision should be delayed, https:// www.kevinmd.com/blog/2020/12/why-male-circumcision-should-be-delayed.html.

808 Piontek, Elizabeth A., Albani, Justin M. Male Circumcision: The Clinical Implications Are More Than Skin Deep. *Mo Med*. Jan-Feb 2019; 116(1):35–37.

809 Edwards, Catherine. Jews and Muslims in Sweden outraged over call to ban male circumcision. *thelocal*, https://www.thelocal.se/20191002/jews-and-muslims-in-sweden -outraged-over-call-to-ban-male-circumcision.

810 Freeman, M. D. A child's right to circumcision. *BJU Int*. Jan 1999; 83 Suppl 1:74–78, https://doi.org/10.1046/j.1464-410x.1999.0830s1074.x.

811 Petrini, Carlo. Ethical and legal considerations regarding the ownership and commercial use of human biological materials and their derivatives. *J Blood Med*. 2012; 3:87–96, https://doi.org/10.2147/JBM.S36134.

812 Skloot, Rebecca. *The Immortal Life of Henrietta Lacks, Skloot, Rebecca.* Crown; 2021. p. 12, https://amazon.com/Immortal-Life-Henrietta-Lacks-ebook/dp/B00338QENI /ref=sr_1_1?crid=1H3DIWGL3M4AT&dchild=1&keywords=the+immortal+life +of+henrietta+lacks+by+rebecca+skloot&qid=1623613155&sprefix=the+immortal +life+%2Caps%2C220&sr=8-1.

813 Calfas, Jennifer. Family of Henrietta Lacks, Whose Unique Cells Changed Science, Settles With Thermo Fisher. *The Wall Street Journal*, https://www.wsj.com/articles /henrietta-lacks-family-hela-cells-thermo-fisher-settlement-d93e60e5.

814 Michael A. Heller, James Salzman. *Mine!: How the Hidden Rules of Ownership Control Our Lives.* Doubleday; 2021. loc. 2889, https://amazon.com/Mine-Hidden-Rules -Ownership-Control-ebook/dp/B08B5F7NNY/ref=sr_1_1?dchild=1&keywords=Mi ne%21%3A+How+the+Hidden+Rules+of+Ownership+Control+Our+Lives&qid =1623612641&sr=8-1.

815 Michael A. Heller, James Salzman. *Mine!: How the Hidden Rules of Ownership Control Our Lives—Kindle edition by Heller, Michael A., Salzman, James. Professional & Technical Kindle eBooks @ Amazon.com.* Doubleday; 2021. loc. 2889.

816 Van Howe, R. S. *Sexual Mutilations: A Human Tragedy.* 1997. Loc. 2879, https:// www.amazon.com/Sexual-Mutilations-Tragedy-Defense-Research-ebook/dp/B000S EPE8Q/ref=sr_1_9?dchild=1&keywords=marilyn+milos&qid=1598373261&sr=8-9.

817 Hood, Leroy, Price, Nathan. *The Age of Scientific Wellness: Why the Future of Medicine Is Personalized, Predictive, Data-Rich, and in Your Hands.* Belknap Press; 2023. loc. 995, https://www.amazon.com/dp/B0BRQRBT7J

818 Circumcision, American Academy of Pediatrics Task Force on. Circumcision policy statement. *Pediatrics.* 2012; 130(3):585–586, https://doi.org/10.1542/peds.2012-1989.

819 Scribd. CDC Proposal On Male Circumcision: December 2, 2014, https://www .scribd.com/document/248978688/CDC-proposal-on-male-circumcision-December -2-2014#scribd.

820 Zuckerman, Wendy. *Circumcision-why are we doing this?* Science Vs. Podcast. 5-31-18, https://gimletmedia.com/shows/science-vs/dvhe5l/circumcision-why-are-we-doing -this.

821 Toviah Garber, Shemuel. *The Circular Cut: Problematizing the Longevity of Civilization's Most Aggressively Defended Amputation.* Wesleyan University; 2013, https://www.academia.edu/4589882/The_Circular_Cut_Problematizing_the_ Longevity_of_Civilization_s_Most_Aggressively_Defended_Amputation.

822 Earp, Brian D. Do the Benefits of Male Circumcision Outweigh the Risks? A Critique of the Proposed CDC Guidelines. *Front Pediatr.* 2015; 3:18, https://doi.org/10.3389 /fped.2015.00018.

823 European docs criticize US support for circumcision. *The Times of Israel.* March 20, 2023, https://www.timesofisrael.com/european-docs-criticize-us-support-for -circumcision/#:~:text=In%20the%20academy's%20report%2C%20the,for%20 surgery%20before%20boys%20are.

824 Blank, Susan, Brady, Michael, et al. Circumcision Policy Statement. *Pediatrics.* 2023; 130(3):585–586, https://doi.org/10.1542/peds.2012-1989.

825 Makary, Marty. *The Price We Pay: What Broke American Health Care—and How to Fix It*. Bloomsbury Publishing; 2019. loc. 3320, https://www.amazon.com/dp /B07MXPJ33B.

826 Dekker, Rebecca. *Babies Are Not Pizzas: They're Born, Not Delivered*. Evidence Based Birth: 2019. p. 101, https://www.amazon.com/gp/product/B07WQGZ695/ref= ppx_yo_dt_b_search_asin_title?ie=UTF8&psc=1.

827 Van Howe, R. S. *Sexual Mutilations: A Human Tragedy*. 1997. Loc. 2879, https:// www.amazon.com/Sexual-Mutilations-Tragedy-Defense-Research-ebook/dp/B000S EPE8Q/ref=sr_1_9?dchild=1&keywords=marilyn+milos&qid=1598373261&sr=8-9.

828 Harryman, Gary. An Analysis of the Accuracy of the Presentation of the Human Penis in Anatomical Source Materials. 2004.

829 Roberts, A. *The Complete Human Body*. DK publishing; 2010.

830 Michael Rovito, Razan Maxson. *Men's Health: An Introduction*. 2020, https:// amazon.com/Mens-Health-Introduction-Diana-Karczmarczyk-ebook/dp/B08BVXV 3S3/ref=sr_1_1?dchild=1&keywords=men%27s+health%3A+an+introduction +milstein&qid=1593874433&sr=8-1.

831 Rachel E. Simon, Noah Grigni. *The Every Body Book: The LGBTQ+ Inclusive Guide for Kids about Sex, Gender, Bodies, and Families*. Jessica Kingsley Publishers; Illustrated edition (June 18, 2020); 2021, https://amazon.com/Every-Body-Book -Inclusive-Families/dp/1787751732/ref=sr_1_1?crid=S9US4T1WNCRO&dchild =1&keywords=the+every+body+book&qid=1625934401&sprefix=the+every+%2 Caps%2C253&sr=8-1.

832 Roach, Mary. *Bonk: The Curious Coupling of Science and Sex*. Reprint edition (April 6, 2009), W. W. Norton & Company; 2009. p. 41.

833 Kalcev, B. Circumcision and personal hygiene in school boys. *Medical Officer*, 112, 171–173. 1964; 112:171–173.

834 Osborn, L. M., Metcalf, T. J., Mariani, E. M. Hygienic care in uncircumcised infants. *Pediatrics*. Mar 1981; 67(3):365–7.

835 Osborn, L. M., Metcalf, T. J., Mariani, E. M. Hygienic care in uncircumcised infants. *Pediatrics*. Mar 1981; 67(3):365–7.

836 Bollinger, Dan. The Penis-Care Information Gap: Preventing Improper Care of Intact Boys. *Thymos: Journal of Boyhood Studies*. 2007/07/01; 1:205–219, https://doi.org /10.3149/thy.0205.219.

837 Narvaez, Darcia. Doctor Ignorance of Male Anatomy Harms Boys. Blog. 2011, http:// www.psychologytoday.com/blog/moral-landscapes/201110/doctor-ignorance-male -anatomy-harms-boys.

838 Liu, Neha, et al. Frequency and Variability of Advice Given to Parents on Care of the Uncircumcised Penis by Pediatric Residents: A Need to Improve Education— Urology. *Pediatric Urology*. 2020; 136:218–224, https://doi.org/doi:10.1016/j.urology .2019.09.057.

839 Gemma Sutton, Samantha Fryer, Grace Rimmer, Charlotte V. Melling, Harriet J. Corbett. Referrals from primary care with foreskin symptoms: Room for improve-ment. *Journal of Pediatric Surgery*. 2023; https://doi.org/10.1016/j.jpedsurg.2022.10 .046.

840 Wodwaski, N., Munyan, K. As nurses, are we meeting the unique needs of the intact client? *J Spec Pediatr Nurs.* Aug 25, 2021:e12356, https://doi.org/10.1111/jspn.12356.

841 Pediatrics, American Academy of. Care of the Uncircumcised Penis. *Pediatric Patient Education.* 2024; https://doi.org/10.1542/peo_document108.

842 Intact America. National Survey Highlights. 2023, https://patch.com/georgia/roswell/calendar/event/20240220/1cbe5a7b-090f-4de4-a535-854998046413/new-memoirs-from-atlanta-s-lucid-house-publishing-will-change-how-america-thinks-about-circumcision.

843 RADIOLAB. *Dispatch 2: Every day is Ignaz Semmelweis Day.* Podcast. April 1, 2020.

844 Saria, Dr. Suchi. *Using AI to Help Doctors Save Lives.* What's Your Problem. February 15, 2024, https://pca.st/pokvhwmo.

845 Van Howe, R. S. *Sexual Mutilations: A Human Tragedy.* 1997. Loc. 2879, https://www.amazon.com/Sexual-Mutilations-Tragedy-Defense-Research-ebook/dp/B000SEPE8Q/ref=sr_1_9?dchild=1&keywords=marilyn+milos&qid=1598373261&sr=8-9.

846 Makary, Marty. *The Price We Pay: What Broke American Health Care—and How to Fix It.* Bloomsbury Publishing; 2019. loc. 3320, https://www.amazon.com/dp/B07MXPJ33B.

847 Earp, Brian David, https://x.com/briandavidearp/status/1721095242693144975.

848 Bonobo3D. Circumcision and Sexual Function Difficulties. YouTube, https://www.youtube.com/watch?v=yfGkZZ-KzpU&list=PLKuasLinBzLvg-s777BUtAX23LTdDfU6g&index=8&t=425s.

849 Morris, Brian J., Krieger, John N. Does male circumcision affect sexual function, sensitivity, or satisfaction?—a systematic review. *J Sex Med.* 2013; 10(11):2644–2657, https://doi.org/10.1111/jsm.12293.

850 Earp, Brian David, https://x.com/briandavidearp/status/1078529309478838272.

851 Briggs, Anne. *Circumcision: What Every Parent Should Know.* Virginia: Birth and Parenting Publications; 2020, https://books.google.com/books/about/Circumcision.html?id=Ll5QHIpNxV8C.

852 Stang, H. J., Snellman, L. W. Circumcision practice patterns in the United States. *Pediatrics.* Jun 1998; 101(6):E5, https://doi.org/10.1542/peds.101.6.e5.

853 Waldenberg, Rabbi Eliezer. *Tzitz Eliezer.* 1950. p. 29.

854 Cooper, Eitan. *Milah Confronts Modernity: Analyzing Debates Over Circumcision Technique.* Brandeis University; 2012. p. 89.

855 Stang, H. J., Snellman, L. W. Circumcision practice patterns in the United States. *Pediatrics.* Jun 1998; 101(6):E5, https://doi.org/10.1542/peds.101.6.e5.

856 Kurtis, Peter S., DeSilva, Hema N., Bernstein, Bruce A., Malakh, Lillian, Schechter, Neil L. A Comparison of the Mogen and Gomco Clamps in Combination With Dorsal Penile Nerve Block in Minimizing the Pain of Neonatal Circumcision. *Pediatrics.* 1999; 103(2):e23-e23, https://doi.org/10.1542/peds.103.2.e23.

857 Margulis, Jennifer. *The Business of Baby.* Scribner, A Division of Simon & Schuster, Inc.; 2013. p. 133.

858 Cooper, Eitan. *Milah Confronts Modernity: Analyzing Debates Over Circumcision Technique.* Brandeis University; 2012. p. 89.

859 Al-Marhoon, M. S., Jaboub, S. M. Plastibell Circumcision: How Safe is it?: Experience at Sultan Qaboos University Hospital. *Sultan Qaboos Univ Med J.* Jun 2006; 6(1):17–20.

860 Emeka, Chukwubuike Kevin. Neonatal circumcision: profile of neonates with complications resulting from the use of plastibell. 2021.

861 Hamza, Babatunde K., Ahmed, Muhammed, Bello, Ahmad, et al. Comparison of the efficacy and safety of circumcision by freehand technique and Plastibell device in children. *African Journal of Urology.* 2020/11/16; 26(1):66, https://doi.org/10.1186 /s12301-020-00076-z.

862 Stang, H. J., Snellman, L. W. Circumcision practice patterns in the United States. *Pediatrics.* Jun 1998; 101(6):E5, https://doi.org/10.1542/peds.101.6.e5.

863 X. D. Jin, J. J. Lu W. H. Liu, et al. Adult male circumcision with a circular stapler versus conventional circumcision: A prospective randomized clinical trial. *Braz J Med res.* 2015.

864 Susan Terkel, Lorna Greenberg. *The Circumcision Decision: An Unbiased Guide for Parents.* Carrot Seed Publishing LLC; 2012. loc. 302.

865 Huang, Pei-Lin, Lee, I. Ching, Tsai, De-Chan, Tsai, Jen-Ho, Tsai, Vincent F. S., Pong, Yuan-Hung. Use of Holmium YAG laser in circumcision: A novel, less complicated and alternative procedure for adolescent. *African Journal of Urology.* 2020/11/17; 26(1):64, https://doi.org/10.1186/s12301-020-00077-y.

866 Abid, Ammar, Hussein, Naser. Meatal stenosis posttraditional neonatal circumcision-cross-sectional study. Original Article. *Urology Annals.* January 1, 2021; 13(1):62–66, https://doi.org/10.4103/ua.Ua_30_20.

867 UNAIDS, Joint United Nations Programme on HIV/AIDS. 2012. Neonatal and child male circumcision: A global review (World Health Organization) (2012).

868 Cooper, Eitan. *Milah Confronts Modernity: Analyzing Debates Over Circumcision Technique.* Brandeis University; 2012. p. 89.

869 Doctors Opposing Circumcision blog, https://www.doctorsopposingcircumcision .org/about-us/#statement-principles.

www.ingramcontent.com/pod-product-compliance
Lightning Source LLC
Chambersburg PA
CBHW051311120626
46547CB00015B/2181